Nerve-Sparing Radical Hysterectomy

Yoshihiko Yabuki

Nerve-Sparing Radical Hysterectomy

English Translation By Shimpachiro Ogiwara & Sandra M Ogiwara

Springer

Yoshihiko Yabuki
Department of Obstetrics and Gynecology
Kanazawa Medical University,
Uchinada, Ishikawa, Japan

International School of Surgical Anatomy
IRCCS Sacro Cuore Don Calabria Hospital
Verona, Italy

ISBN 978-981-96-7193-9 ISBN 978-981-96-7194-6 (eBook)
https://doi.org/10.1007/978-981-96-7194-6

This Springer imprint is published by the registered company Springer Nature Singapore Pte Ltd.
The registered company address is: 152 Beach Road, #21-01/04 Gateway East, Singapore 189721, Singapore

Preface

Today's surgery for cervical cancer can be roughly categorized into simple total hysterectomy, Wertheim surgery, nerve-sparing radical hysterectomy (NSRH), and Latzko/Okabayashi/Meigs surgery. However, while NSRH is recognized in the literature in the West, it is not commonly carried out as a routine procedure. Furthermore, the Latzko/Okabayashi/Meigs procedures do not meet today's quality of life except in special cases. Therefore, in the West, the surgical options for FIGO stage I cervical cancer are limited to a simple total hysterectomy and the Wertheim or modified Wertheim procedure. For patients whose stage of cancer necessitates NSRH, concurrent chemoradiotherapy is carried out. The current situation in distinction between Wertheim surgery and NSRH remains very blurred, raising strong concerns that the latter may be phased out from cervical cancer surgery.

The history of NSRH developed in parallel to concurrent discoveries of new anatomic theories and techniques. For example, Savage/Kocks' cardinal ligament (CL; a bundle between the uterine cervix and ureter) gave birth to the Wertheim procedure, and Mackenrodt's transverse cervical ligament (TCL; a bundle connecting the uterine cervix to the pelvic sidewall) to the Latzko/Okabayashi procedure. These twentieth-century hysterectomy procedures were based on gross/systematic anatomy, or basic anatomy. However, the anatomy required in today's surgery is clinical anatomy, which gives a means of describing surgically created artifacts such as CL and TCL. An ongoing challenge in cervical cancer surgery is the lack of a clear distinction between these two artifacts, evident in the understanding of "the cardinal ligament of Mackenrodt," which is reflected in surgical techniques.

The parametrium proposed by the author, which is based on clinical anatomy, consists of the following: (1) a horizontal continuum composed of the uterine broad ligament, "the condensation in the base of the broad ligament," or CL, and paracolpium; (2) a perpendicular continuum, or supporting system, composed of the vesicohypogastric fascia, TCL, and lateral rectal ligament; (3) a vaso-neural lamina, or mesoureter, attached to the dorsal aspect of the ureter, which includes the posterior layer of Okabayashi's vesicouterine ligament, or the anterior mesoureter; and (4) a longitudinal continuum, or suspensory system, consisting of the uterosacral ligament, cervical fascia, and pubocervical ligament, including the bladder pillar and anterior layer of Okabayashi's vesicouterine ligament. The author's lateral parametrectomy, which is based on the above, involves creating four spaces around the intersection of TCL and the mesoureter, selectively excising connective tissue and blood vessels from the separated ligaments/laminae. Notably, intraoperative hemorrhaging in this procedure was significantly reduced by non-excision of the lateral rectal ligament with preservation of bladder function achieved by excising only the superior vesical vein, or the vein connecting the bladder to the deep uterine vein, from the isolated anterior mesoureter.

Presently, equal access to HPV vaccine or chemoradiotherapy is not available worldwide. Furthermore, current anticancer drugs have not sufficiently progressed to a level that would render surgical treatment of cervical cancer obsolete. The author hopes this book promotes the practice of NSRH and preserves it as a surgical legacy for the twenty-first century until advances in vaccines and drug therapy eliminate the need for surgical intervention.

Kanazawa, Ishikawa, Japan Yoshihiko Yabuki

Acknowledgments

The compilation of this book on RH was made possible by the collaboration of many colleagues and hospital staff at Ishikawa Prefectural Central Hospital. Furthermore, the author would like to express his heartfelt gratitude to Dr. Gen Murakami MD, PhD, former professor of anatomy at Sapporo Medical University, for his guidance in human anatomic dissections, and to Dr. Shimpachiro Ogiwara, PT, SRP(UK), ONC(UK), CPA(C), BPT(C), MA(USA), PhD(USA), former professor at the University of Kanazawa, and his wife Sandra, MCPA(UK), HT(UK), CPA(C), BScPT(C), for undertaking English translation of this work since 1991 until the publication of this book. The author is deeply grateful to Takayuki Enomoto, MD, PhD, and Mikio Mikami, MD, PhD, former professors at the University of Niigata and Tokai University, respectively, for their kind cooperation in publishing this book. In addition, the author extends his heartfelt thanks to Mr. Hidenori Maeda, CEO of Maeda Shoten, Co, Ltd, and Ms. Saki Kasai of Springer Nature Japan for their assistance in this endeavor.

With the deepest of gratitude, this book is dedicated to my late wife, Eiko, who had supported me tirelessly throughout my entire professional career (Yabuki 2022).

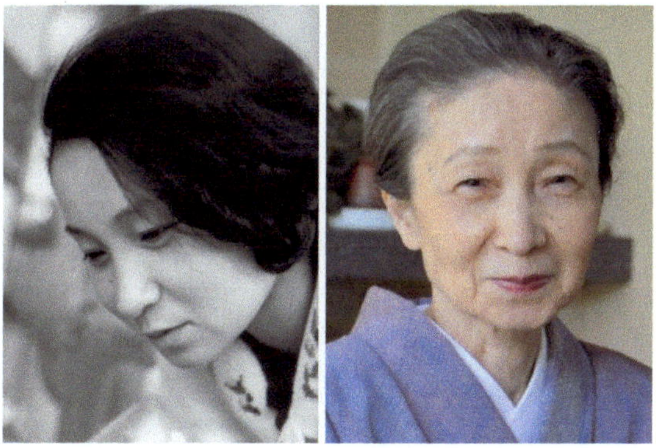

Portrait of my late wife (Yabuki 2022)

Reference

Yabuki Y (2022) Homage to my wife: life lived during conception and development of surgical procedure for uterine cervical cancer. Maeda Shoten, Kanazawa. (in Japanese)

Contents

Chapter 1
Introduction

Abbreviations

CL	Cardinal ligament
IFFA	International Federation of Associations of Anatomists
IHP	Inferior hypogastric plexus
L&S	Latzko and Schiffmann
LP	Lateral parametrium
LUL	Lateral umbilical ligament
NSRH	Nerve-sparing radical hysterectomy
P&A	Peham-Americh
PSN	Pelvic splanchnic nerve
Q&M	Querleu and Morrow
RH	Radical hysterectomy
TA	Terminologia Anatomica
TCL	Transverse cervical ligament
TMMR	Total mesometrial resection
VUL	Vesicouterine ligament

1 Background

Throughout the world's gynecological circles, the definition of radical hysterectomy (RH) remains ambiguous. In the West, the Wertheim or modified Wertheim procedure is principally carried out (Ramirez et al. 2018; Plante et al. 2024), whereas in East Asia, RH is centered on a modified Okabayashi procedure, that is, preservation of the lateral rectal ligament and vesical nerve branches (Yabuki et al. 1991, 1996, 2000; Yabuki 1997). The differences between the two principal surgical procedures in these geographical zones are primarily one of excision or non-excision of the deep uterine vein and its surrounding connective tissue and whether or not the vesical nerve branches are intentionally preserved.

Y. Yabuki, *Nerve-Sparing Radical Hysterectomy*,
https://doi.org/10.1007/978-981-96-7194-6_1

In general, surgery for cancer of the uterine cervix consists of a simple hysterectomy, Wertheim procedure (Wertheim 1911, 1912), nerve-sparing radical hysterectomy (NSRH) (Yabuki et al. 1991, 1996, 2000; Yabuki 1997), and Latzko/Okabayashi/Meigs procedure (Latzko and Schiffmann 1919; Okabayashi 1921, 1952; Meigs 1954) where each procedure carried out is dependent on the stage of cancer. However, NSRH in the West still remains a surgical procedure that exists only in the literature and has not been generalized nor reached clinical trials (Ramirez et al. 2018; Plante et al. 2024; Querleu and Morrow 2008; Cibula et al. 2011; Magrina et al. 2011). The history of surgery for cancer of the uterine cervix in the West has not progressed from the Wertheim and Latzko/Meigs procedures, and the deficiency between these two procedures is compensated currently by concurrent chemoradiotherapy (CCRT) (Morris et al. 1999; Rose et al. 1999). According to the author's experience, the prognosis for surgical treatment, especially NSRH and/or Meigs procedure, depends greatly on the surgeon's technical skill, and it may be impossible to analyze the outcome for a large population of patients for chemoradiotherapy (CRT). To solve this problem, it would require a meta-analysis involving a randomized controlled trial (RCT) on small groups of patients operated on by highly skilled surgeons, but this has not yet been implemented. The *raison d'être* for surgery lies in it being an additional treatment to CRT. Whether this additional treatment encompasses the Wertheim procedure or NSRH has not yet been decided. However, if one adheres to the Western treatment policy, extinction of NSRH as a choice of surgery for the uterine cervix will certainly be a possibility in the future.

Decrease in intraoperative hemorrhaging and preservation of bladder and rectal function had long been an earnest wish for gynecologic surgeons. A successful surgery far outweighs the side effects of chemotherapy and/or radiotherapy. Moreover, NSRH with a minimally invasive technique may help surgeons discover new surgical procedures and anatomy. From this perspective, RH must be continued.

2 Goal of This Book

This book based on anatomy and histology was undertaken to establish surgical techniques for RH, conforming to a twenty-first century quality of life (QOL). The author has earnestly pursued this endeavor since the latter half of the twentieth century. Furthermore, the author wishes this book to be preserved for posterity as a surgical heritage of this century, which would be comparable to the Latzko/Okabayashi procedure of the twentieth century. This publication focuses on the following five perspectives.

2.1 *Characteristics of Radical Hysterectomy in the Twentieth Century*

Procedure for RH of the twentieth century was initiated and established by Latzko & Schiffmann (L&S) (1919), and Okabayashi (1921, 1952) who pursued extensive excision for curative purposes. Their surgical procedure involved the separation and resection of the transverse cervical ligament (TCL) (Mackenrodt 1895; Speert 1996), that is, a bundle connecting the cervix and pelvic sidewall, at the pelvic floor. However, this procedure was associated with significant shortcomings such as massive hemorrhage and functional impairments in adjacent organs. The distinction between the L&S and Okabayashi procedures was their difference in opinion principally concerning the vesicouterine ligament. In the West, the Wertheim procedure is more frequently used as an alternative, involving excision of the cardinal ligament, or *CL* (Savage 1870; Kocks 1880), that is, a bundle connecting the ureter and uterine cervix, rather than TCL. This procedure is frequently referred to as a modified Wertheim operation (Averette et al. 1993; Meigs 1945; Höckel et al. 2003) and involves excavation of the paravesical and pararectal spaces, but in many cases, excision of the deep uterine vein is not specified. Of course, the handling of the posterior layer of Okabayashi's vesicouterine ligament, or *anterior mesoureter* (Okabayashi 1952; Hoshiba et al. 2000; Yabuki et al. 2005), is entirely outside the scope of the modified Wertheim procedure. The vesical nerve branch is also never mentioned in this surgical procedure. Höckel's total mesometrial resection (TMMR) (Höckel et al. 2003), which incorporates ontogenetic anatomy, can be considered a representative variation. In Japan, this procedure is referred to as a semi-RH to distinguish it from an RH. Therefore, the author harbors some doubts regarding the surgical outcomes of RH in the West. In contrast, RH carried out in Asia primarily follows Yabuki's NSRH (Yabuki et al. 1991, 1996, 2000, 2005, 2011; Yabuki 1997, 2007, 2016, 2019, 2020; Hoshiba et al. 2000), that is, a modification of the Okabayashi procedure.

2.2 *The Author's Surgical Experience: Past and Present—With Radical Hysterectomy*

The author commenced the Okabayashi procedure in 1980 but struggled with intraoperative hemorrhaging and postoperative bladder dysfunction. To address these issues, thorough excision of the ligaments and their associated blood vessels using the cavitron ultrasonic surgical aspirator (CUSA), followed by lymphadenectomy, was carried out. Hemorrhaging was resolved by the preservation of the lateral rectal ligament (AJOG; 1991), while bladder dysfunction was alleviated by preserving the vesical nerve branch (Gynecol Oncol; 1996). Based on anatomic knowledge gained during this period, the author in the year 2000 successfully carried out the entire process for laparoscopic NSRH, and this surgical procedure was verified by simulated RH on fresh cadavers (AJOG; 2005 (Yabuki et al. 2005)). This study was conducted at the Sapporo Medical University, Department of Anatomy, under the guidance of former Professor Murakami from the year 2000 to 2003. A part of this achievement was published in an article titled "Discrepancies between classic anatomy and modern gynecologic surgery on pelvic connective tissue structure: harmonization of those concepts by collaborative cadaver dissection" (Hill 2020) in AJOG. The following is a comment from the editor regarding this chapter:

Commentary *The face of medical education has changed dramatically in the past decade. For medical students all the way to practicing physician, information transfer has evolved from pedantic lectures to include on-line program with virtual patients, interactive seminars with hand-on models, and hired actors trained as "professional" patients. Students at all stages must still ultimately…study! The authors of this article report classical anatomical observation; reminding us that anatomy is the crux of surgery. This carful dissection of the female pelvis illustrates the relationships between the vital structures and major vessels. As more pelvic surgeons begin to use procedures such as blind needle insertion of tapes and support materials, a mental image of these relationships may help eschew injury. The authors thoughtfully point out that as our surgical armamentarium expands, it is always worthwhile to review the basic principles we learned at the cadaver.*

The author's past experience with the Okabayashi procedure evolved into a nerve-sparing extended RH (Yabuki 2019). So, the shortcomings of twentieth century RH have largely been addressed, but the author's surgical techniques are regrettably seldom discussed in the literature. This can be inferred from the fact that many articles describe the use of Piver's classification class III (Piver et al. 1974) in contemporary surgical procedure for cervical cancer. Piver class III corresponds to Meigs surgery (Meigs 1954), which involves excision of the lateral rectal ligament. Fortunately, the circumstances at the time began to demand minimally invasive surgery, which coincided with the introduction of laparoscopic-assisted RH and the publication of articles by Querleu in 1991 and Nezhat in 1993 on laparoscopic pelvic lymphadenectomy (Querleu et al. 1991; Nezhat et al. 1993). The proposed author's laparoscopic-assisted RH based on cadaver dissection in 2000 coincided with and met the demands of the time.

2.3 Discussion on Controversial Terminology in Anatomy

Until the latter half of the twentieth century, gynecologists only had the means of basic anatomy to describe artifacts resulting from surgical manipulations. There was, up until that time, historically and traditionally too great a disparity in academia between gynecologic surgery and anatomy for surgeons to face the challenge of the anatomists. Furthermore, many idiomatically expressed terms in clinical practice, such as the vesicouterine ligament, cardinal ligament, and uterosacral ligament, often lacked scientifically based definitions. Moreover, a significant number of clinical terms even today still rely on late nineteenth-century clinical anatomy by Savage (1870), Kocks (1880), and Mackenrodt (1895). Furthermore, RH always remains in a state of flux, bringing changes in the definition of terms as surgical procedures progress. Therefore, the relationship is likely to remain ambiguous between the basic and clinical anatomies.

Under such circumstances, gynecologists have endeavored to reconcile this divergence between theory, or *anatomy*, and practice, or *surgery*, although only through their surgical techniques. As a result, the understanding of changes in the morphology caused by surgical intervention in RH has diverged significantly from that of basic anatomy and that of anatomy conceived by gynecological sciences (Yabuki et al. 1991, 1996, 2000; Yabuki 1997; Wertheim 1911, 1912; Latzko and Schiffmann 1919; Okabayashi 1921; Peham and Amreich 1930, 1934; Uhlenhuth et al. 1948; Reiffenstuhl 1982; Clemente 1985). To address this issue, the International Federation of Associations of Anatomists announced in 1998 that idiomatic clinical terms such as TCL be introduced in Terminologia Anatomica (Drake et al. 2005). Basic anatomy practiced by anatomists is considered a discipline aimed at representing the human body as faithfully as possible in its natural state. However, if one were to ask the anatomist the question of whether artificially manipulated forms of the body constitute anatomy, many would most likely disagree. In contrast, clinical anatomy as described by the author is a means of explaining clinically created artifacts. For example, Gray's Anatomy for Students (Williams and Warwick 1980), first published in 2005, included illustrations of the uterosacral ligament, TCL, and pubocervical ligament (Williams and Warwick 1980; Fig. 5.57). This marked the first occurrence of such illustrations in the history of Gray's Anatomy. However, if one were to ask gynecologists whether an illustration portraying the subserous layer as a continuous fascia is beneficial to surgery, many would likely disagree, because it is composed of ligaments that exist in pairs, corresponding to multiple spaces. Furthermore, the term "the cardinal ligament (of Mackenrodt)" (Uhlenhuth et al. 1948; Reiffenstuhl 1982) has been used since around the 1940s. But the 36th British edition of Gray's Anatomy in 1980 disregarded this term in its historical contributions to RH, referring to it as TCL of Mackenrodt (Mackenrodt 1895; Speert 1996). This led to confusion in the boundaries between the Latzko/Okabayashi/Meigs and Wertheim procedures. The author is therefore concerned that premature surgery or clinical anatomy may perpetuate clearly defined basic anatomy as an ambiguous discipline (Yabuki et al. 1991).

2.4 Basic Anatomy and Clinical Anatomy

While carrying out simulated RH on fresh cadavers, the author keenly felt that, to accurately describe surgical procedure precisely, there was a need for surgery-specific anatomic terms. At the same time, he realized the impossibility of classifying three-dimensional structures altered by surgical manipulation based solely on two-dimensional cross-sectioned images of pelvic organs as demonstrated by Querleu and Morrow (Q&M) (2008). The author believed that new clinical terms were required to describe these three-dimensional structures.

Ramanah and DeLancy et al. (2012) stated in 2012 that it is possible to analyze pelvic ligaments in women by 3D MRI imaging. In addition, another requirement surgeons wish for is a way to describe the deformed morphology when an artifact, such as a space, is created in the body during surgery. An article by DeLancy et al. (1992) in 1992 depicted the paracolpium as a bundle directly connecting the vagina and pelvic sidewall in apical or level I support, or *suspension*. According to the author's observation and experience in carrying out the Okabayashi procedure and through cadaver dissection, the paracolpium and the superior fascia of the pelvic diaphragm can be considered a continuum of TCL and the lateral rectal ligament. Could it be that this proposal by DeLancy et al., which is based on basic anatomic concepts, lacks surgical observation? Moreover, in their 2012 analysis of the 3D MRI images, they should have examined the relationship between ligaments and adjacent organs.

Unfortunately, in the field of gynecology, gastroenterology, and urology, surgeons have come to no mutual understanding on clinical terminology including its concepts; consequently, it is rarely used as a common language in these fields. This indicates the underdevelopment of research in pelvic anatomy in its relationship to pelvic surgery and remains an important issue to be considered in the future. One potential solution lies in the significant advancements in diagnostic body imaging techniques. Indeed, collaborative research starting from the stage of ontogenetic anatomy could prove very beneficial.

This book is based on the author's research, knowledge, and experience of the anatomy and surgical procedures carried out for cervical cancer inherited from the nineteenth and twentieth centuries. The author has attempted to demonstrate the potentiality of clinical anatomy independent from basic anatomy primarily focused on its application to surgery together with a scholarly coexistence and integration.

2.5 Proposal for and Expectation of Twenty-First Century Radical Hysterectomy

By the end of the twentieth century, research and efforts in treatment of cervical cancer were directed toward the introduction of chemoradiotherapy and human papilloma virus (HPV) vaccination (Morris et al. 1999; Rose et al. 1999; Garland et al. 2016; Kjaer et al. 2021), with the aim of avoiding surgical risks as well as toward the implementation of cervical cancer screening (Machii and Saito 2011; Hill 2020). Fortunately, these developments led to a reduction in the number of surgical cases, but this led to a decrease in opportunities for gynecological surgeons to acquire technical skills (Matsuo et al. 2021). To compensate for this lack of technical proficiency, there has been a trend toward simplification and/or omission of procedures without any accompanying anatomic theory (Cibula et al. 2011). This situation raises concerns about the loss of curative intent. In other words, concurrent chemoradiotherapy (CCRT) (Morris et al. 1999; Rose et al. 1999; Green et al. 2001; Monk et al. 2023; Rallis et al. 2021) is being emphasized in the West, and surgery is being limited to Wertheim surgery or modified Wertheim surgery (Querleu and Morrow 2008; Cibula et al. 2011; Magrina et al. 2011; Averette et al. 1993; Meigs 1945, 1950; Höckel et al. 2003) ,with surgical cases increasingly restricted to early-stage cancer.

In their classification published in 2008, Q&M included NSRH, or type C1 Operation (Querleu and Morrow 2008), and in 2011, along with Cibula et al., added non-excision of the deep uterine vein to the type C1 Operation (Cibula et al. 2011). Furthermore, an article was accepted by the New England Journal of Medicine indicating no statistical distinction in prognosis between patients who had undergone Ramirez et al.'s Piver class II operation (Ramirez et al. 2018), or Wertheim surgery (Wertheim 1912; Piver et al. 1974), and that by Piver class III operation, or Meigs surgery. (Wertheim 1912; Meigs 1954)

It is most likely that with time, laparoscopic/robot-assisted RH, or *minimally invasive surgery*, and open abdominal RH will reach the same level of proficiency. However, even if both surgeries reach the same technical level, if they continue to adhere to the technique of not excising the deep uterine vein as performed by Q&M and Cibula et al. (2011), or the technique described by Ramirez et al (Yabuki 2023), that is, Wertheim surgery or semi-RH, true radicality may not be attained and passed down to future surgeons. This trend raises concerns about the loss of traditional or true RH, which involves complete excision of TCL.

Unfortunately, in the world today, there are still many facilities not sufficiently equipped for radiation therapy. According to the Global Cancer Observatory Report (Bray et al. 2018) in 2018, the age-standardized rates per 100,000 for cervical cancer incidence/mortality are as follows: 43.1/20.2 in Southern Africa and 40.1/30.0 in Eastern Africa compared to 6.8/2.1 in Western Europe, and 6.4/1.9 in Northern America (Reiffenstuhl 1982). These ratios imply that access to expensive medication and the benefits of CCRT are unavailable to many of these people.

There are cases of cervical cancer, such as non-HPV-related cervical adenocarcinomas, or commonly known as serous carcinomas of the cervix, including gastric-type, clear-cell, mesonephric, and endometrioid adenocarcinomas (Park 2020; Su et al. 2023), where radiation therapy or chemotherapy may be ineffective. Surgery is, in a sense, versatile and an excellent surgeon with anatomy manuals can acquire skills through self-study. Furthermore, it is wise to remember that obstetric accidents such as hemorrhaging will always be a possibility.

It is hard to understand why Okabayashi's posterior layer of the vesicouterine ligament (Okabayashi 1952) is hardly recognized in the West, for the posterior layer contains numerous veins connecting the bladder and TCL as well as the pelvic autonomic nerves. The author has experienced cases during childbirth that appear to have a hematoma in the posterior layer, and in such instances, experience and knowledge of RH has proven to be helpful. It is also true that surgeries for deep endometriosis (Ceccaroni et al. 2012), cervical lesions, and/or intramural fibroids require a high level of skill supported by experience in NSRH.

To pass on RH for future generations, it is necessary to first establish new surgical techniques that meet the current QOL standards. This new surgical approach entails the discovery of cutting-edge procedures (Yabuki et al. 1991, 1996; Latzko and Schiffmann 1919; Okabayashi 1921; Ceccaroni et al. 2012) based on innovative anatomic concepts (Yabuki et al. 1991, 1996; Mackenrodt 1895; Savage 1870). Therefore, it is essential to establish a new anatomy based on knowledge gained from L&S, Okabayashi, and Meigs surgeries and disseminate it as a globally unified new surgical procedure, ideally followed by establishing globally recognized facilities dedicated to intensive surgical training and practice where the surgeon can gain the skills required in a safe learning environment.

The International Federation of Gynecology and Obstetrics (FIGO) does not recognize surgical treatment for stage IIB cervical cancer. However, one of the factors determining the surgical outcome of cervical cancer is the presence or absence of lymph node metastasis. It is predicted that if future anticancer drugs are effective against lymph node metastasis, the applicability of surgery may be valued more than it is now. Indeed, the progress in HPV vaccines and drug therapy will eventually lead to the eradication of cervical cancer. A perfected NSRH of the twenty-first century must be preserved as a surgical legacy even if the time arrives when NSRH is no longer necessary just as the historical surgical legacies left behind by L&S and Okabayashi. The author publishes this humble book on gynecologic surgery with the hope of contributing, albeit in a small way, to that legacy.

Abbreviations used in this book are presented as follows: a: artery, a&v: artery and vein, lig: ligament, v: vein, CL: cardinal ligament, IFAA: International Federation of Associations of Anatomists, L&S: Latzko and Schiffmann, NSRH: nerve-sparing radical hysterectomy, P&A: Peham-Amreich, Q&M: Querleu and Morrow, RH: radical hysterectomy, TCL: transverse cervical ligament, TMMR: total mesometrial resection. P&A's diagrams are from Gynäkologische Operationslehre (P&A 1930) and modified by the author.

References

Averette HE, Nguyen HN, Donato DM et al (1993) Radical hysterectomy for invasive cervical cancer: a 25-year prospective experience with the Miami technique. Cancer Suppl 71:1422–1437. PMID: 8431876. https://doi.org/10.1002/cncr.2820710407

Bray F, Ferlay J, Soerjomataram I et al (2018) Global cancer statistics 2018: GLOBOCAN estimates of incidence and mortality worldwide for 36 cancers in 185 countries. CA Cancer J Clin 68(6):394–424. https://doi.org/10.3322/caac.21492

Ceccaroni M, Clarizia R, Bruni F et al (2012) Nerve-sparing laparoscopic eradication of deep endometriosis with segmental rectal and parametrial resection: the Negrar method. A single-center, prospective, clinical trial. Surg Endosc 26:2029–2045. https://doi.org/10.1007/s00464-012-2153-

Cibula D, Abu-Rustum NR, Benedetti-Panici P et al (2011) New classification system of radical hysterectomy: emphasis on a three-dimensional anatomic template for parametrial resection.

Gynecol Oncol 122:264–268. PMID: 21592548. Epub 2011 May 17. https://doi.org/10.1016/j.ygyno.2011.04.029

Clemente CD (ed) (1985) Anatomy of the human body by Henry Gray, 30th American ed, vol 1. Lea & Febiger, Philadelphia, pp 1574–1577

DeLancy JOL (1992) Anatomic aspects of vaginal eversion after hysterectomy. Am J Obstet Gynecol 166:1717–1728. PMID: 1615980. https://doi.org/10.1016/0002-9378(92)91562-o

Drake RL, Vogl W, Mitchell AWM (eds) (2005) Gray's anatomy for students. Elsevier, Philadelphia

Garland SM, Kjaer SK, Muñoz N et al (2016) Impact and effectiveness of the quadrivalent human papillomavirus vaccine: a systematic review of 10 years of real-world experience. Clin Infect Dis 63(4):519–527. PMID:27230391, PMCID: PMC4967609. https://doi.org/10.1093/cid/ciw354

Green JA, Kirwan JM, Tierney JF et al (2001) Survival and recurrence after concomitant chemotherapy and radiotherapy for cancer of the uterine cervix: a systematic review and meta-analysis. Lancet 385:781–786. PMID: 11564482. https://doi.org/10.1016/S0140-6736(01)05965-7

Hill EK (2020) Updates in cervical cancer treatment. Clin Obstet Gynecol 63(1):3–11. https://doi.org/10.1097/GRF.0000000000000507. PMID: 31815773

Höckel M, Horn LC, Hentschel B et al (2003) Total mesometrial resection: high resolution nerve-sparing radical hysterectomy based on developmentally defined surgical anatomy. Int J Gynecol Cancer 13:791–803. PMID: 14675316. https://doi.org/10.1111/j.1525-1438.2003.13608.x

Hoshiba T, Yabuki Y, Asamoto A et al (2000) Our laporoscopic radical hysterectomy. Gynecol Obstet Surg 11:93–100. (in Japanese)

Kjaer SK, Dehlendorff C, Belmonte F et al (2021) Real-world effectiveness of human papilloma virus vaccination against cervical cancer. J Natl Cancer Inst 113(10):1329–1335. https://doi.org/10.1093/jnci/djab080. PMID: 33876216

Kocks J (1880) Die Normale und Pathologische Lage und Gestalt des Uterus Sowie deren Mechanik. Max Cohen & Sohn, Bonn

Latzko W, Schiffmann J (1919) Zur Radikaloperation des Gebarmutterkrebses. 361 Diskussinsbemerkungen. Zbl Gynäk 43:689–698

Machii R, Saito H (2011) Time trends in cervical cancer screening rates in the OECD countries. Jpn J Clin Oncol 41(5):731–732. https://doi.org/10.1093/jjco/hyr058. PMID: 21536695

Mackenrodt A (1895) Ueber die Ursachen der normalen und pathologischen Lagen des Uterus. Arch F Gynäk 48:393–421

Magrina JF, Pawlina W, Kho RM et al (2011) Robotic nerve-sparing radical hysterectomy: feasibility and technique. Gynecol Oncol 121:605–609. PMID: 21419478. https://doi.org/10.1016/j.ygyno.2011.02.034

Matsuo K, Mandelbaum RS, Klar M et al (2021) Decreasing utilization of minimally invasive hysterectomy for cervical cancer in the United States. Gynecol Oncol 162:43–49. PMID: 33992450. https://doi.org/10.1016/j.ygyno.2021.05.005

Meigs JV (1945) Wertheim operation for carcinoma of cervix. Am J Obstet Gynecol 49:542–553

Meigs JV (1950) Radical hysterectomy for cancer of the cervix with bilateral pelvic lymphadenectomy (the so-called Wertheim operation). In: Meigs JV (ed) Progress in gynecology, vol 1. Grune Stratton, New York, pp 540–560

Meigs JV (1954) Radical hysterectomy with bilateral dissection of the pelvic lymph nodes. In: Meigs JV (ed) Surgical treatment of cancer of the cervix. Grune Stratton, New York, pp 149–216

Monk BJ, Toita T, Wu X et al (2023) Durvalumab versus placebo with chemoradiotherapy for locally advanced cervical cancer (CALLA): a randomized, double-blind, phase 3 trial. Lancet Oncol 24(12):1334–1348. https://doi.org/10.1016/S1470-2045(23)00479-5. PMID: 38039991

Morris M, Eifel PJ, Lu J et al (1999) Pelvic radiation with concurrent chemotherapy compared with pelvic and para-aortic radiation for high-risk cervical cancer. N Engl J Med 340:1137–1143. https://doi.org/10.1056/NEJM199904153401501. PMID: 10202164

Nezhat CR, Nezhat FR, Burrell MO (1993) Laparoscopic radical hysterectomy and laparoscopically assisted vaginal radical hysterectomy with pelvic and paraaortic lymph node dissection. J Gynecol Surg 9:105–120. PMID: 10171974. https://doi.org/10.1089/gyn.1993.9.105

Okabayashi H (1921) Radical abdominal hysterectomy for cancer of cervix uteri. Surg Gynecol Obstet 33:335–341

Okabayashi H (1952) Systematic abdominal radical hysterectomy for cancer of cervix uteri. Tokyo, Kanehara (in Japanese)

Park KJ (2020) Cervical adenocarcinoma: integration of HPV status, pattern of invasion, morphology and molecular markers into classification. Histopathology 76(1):112–127. https://doi.org/10.1111/his.13995. PMID: 31846527

Peham HV, Amreich J. (1930) Gynäkologische Operationslehre. Verlag S. Karger, Berlin, Abb 131, 190.

Peham HV, Amreich J (1934) Operative Gynecology, vol. 2 (translated by Ferguson LK). JB Lippincott, Philadelphia, pp 333–366

Piver MS, Rutledge F, Smith JP (1974) Five classes of extended hysterectomy for women with cervical cancer. Obstet Gynecol 44:265–271. PMID: 4417035. [PubMed] [Google Scholar]

Plante M, Kwon JS, Ferguson S, Samouëlian V, Ferron G et al (2024) Simple versus radical hysterectomy in women with low-risk cervical cancer. N Engl J Med 390:819–829. https://doi.org/10.1056/NEJMoa2308900

Querleu D, Morrow CP (2008) Classification of radical hysterectomy. Lancet Oncol 9:297–303. PMID:18308255. https://doi.org/10.1016/S1470-2045(08)70074-3

Querleu D, Leblanc E, Castelain B (1991) Laparoscopic pelvic lymphadenectomy in the early carcinoma of the cervix. Am J Obstet Gynecol 164:579–581. https://doi.org/10.1016/s0002-9378(11)80025-6

Rallis KS, Lai Yau TH, Sideris M (2021) Chemoradiotherapy in cancer treatment: rationale and clinical applications. Anticancer Res 41(1):1–7. https://doi.org/10.21873/anticanres.14746. PMID: 33419794

Ramanah R, Berger MB, Parratte BM et al (2012) Anatomy and histology of apical support: a literature review concerning cardinal and uterosacral ligament. Int Urogynecol J 23:1483–1494. https://doi.org/10.1007/s00192-012-1819-7. PMID: 22618209 PMCID: PMC4258694

Ramirez PT, Frumovitz M, Pareja R et al (2018) Minimally invasive versus abdominal radical hysterectomy for cervical cancer. N Engl J Med 379:1895–1904. PMID: 30380365. https://doi.org/10.1056/NEJMoa1806395

Reiffenstuhl G (1982) The clinical significance of the connective tissue planes and spaces. Clin Obstet Gynecol 25:812–820

Rose PG, Bundy BN, Watkins EB et al (1999) Concurrent cisplatin-based radiotherapy and chemotherapy for locally advanced cervical cancer. N Engl J Med 340:1144–1153. PMID: 10202165. https://doi.org/10.1056/NEJM199904153401502

Savage H (1870) The surgery, surgical pathology, and surgical anatomy of the female pelvic organ, 3rd edn. J & A Churchill & Son, London, p 76

Speert H (1996) Obstetrics and gynecologic milestones illustrated. Parthenon, New York, pp 138–141

Su Y, Zhang Y, Zhou M et al (2023) Genetic alterations in juvenile cervical clear cell adenocarcinoma unrelated to human papillomavirus. Front Med (Lausanne) 16(10):1211888. https://doi.org/10.3389/fmed.2023.1211888.eCollection. PMID: 37654657

Uhlenhuth E, Day DE, Smith RD et al (1948) The visceral endopelvic fascia and the hypogastric sheath. Surg Gynecol Obstet 86:9–28. PMID: 18920874

Wertheim E (1911) Die erweiterte abdominale Operation bei Carcinoma colli uteri (auf Grund von 500 Fällen). Urban & Schwarzenberg, Berlin, pp 356–357

Wertheim E (1912) The extended abdominal operation for carcinoma uteri (based on 500 operative cases). Am J Obstet Dis Women Child 66:169–232

Williams PL, Warwick R (eds) (1980) Gray' anatomy, 36th British ed. Churchill Livingstone, London

Yabuki Y (1997) Cardinal ligament dissection based on a new theory. CEM J Gynecol Oncol 2:278–287. [Google Scholar]

Yabuki Y (2007) Anatomy of the pelvis for radical hysterectomy: does extensive resection of the vagina result in severer bladder dysfunction? The 16th annual review course on gynecologic oncology and pathology. Kyoto, Japan

Yabuki Y (2016) Clinical anatomy of the subserous layer: an amalgamation of gross and clinical anatomy. Clin Anat 29:508–515

Yabuki Y (2019) New radical hysterectomy for uterine cancer, 3rd ed.: theory and technique for nerve-sparing operation. Tokyo: Medical View (in Japanese with figure legend in English)

Yabuki Y (2020) Twenty-first century radical hysterectomy: journey from descriptive to practical anatomy. Gynecol Oncol Rep 34:100623. PMID: 32984492, PMCID: PMC7498749. https://doi.org/10.1016/j.gore.2020.100623

Yabuki Y (2023) Two lateral parametria in radical hysterectomy: history and outcome. J Obstet Gynecol Res 43:1069–1078. https://doi.org/10.1111/jog.15559

Yabuki Y, Asamoto A, Hoshiba T et al (1991) Dissection of the cardinal ligament in radical hysterectomy for cervical cancer with emphasis on the lateral ligament. Am J Obstet Gynecol 164:7–14. PMID: 1986630. https://doi.org/10.1016/0002-9378(91)90614-w

Yabuki Y, Asamoto A, Hoshiba T et al (1996) A new proposal for radical hysterectomy. Gynecol Oncol 62:370–378. PMID: 8812535. [PubMed]. https://doi.org/10.1006/gyno.1996.0251

Yabuki Y, Asamoto A, Hoshiba T et al (2000) Radical hysterectomy: an anatomic evaluation of parametrial dissection. Gynecol Oncol 77:155–163. PMID: 10739705. https://doi.org/10.1006/gyno.1999

Yabuki Y, Sasaki H, Hatakeyama N et al (2005) Discrepancies between classic anatomy and modern gynecologic surgery on pelvic connective tissue structure: harmonization of those concepts by collaborative cadaver dissection. Am J Obstet Gynecol 193:7–15. PMID: 16021052. https://doi.org/10.1016/j.ajog.2005.02.108

Yabuki Y, Murakami G, Hoshiba T et al (2011) Redefinition of the pelvic connective tissue: in-situ histologic examination. Female Pelvic Med Reconstr Surg 17:60–66

Chapter 2
Classical Anatomy and Surgical Procedure

Abbreviations

CL	Cardinal ligament
IFFA	International Federation of Associations of Anatomists
IHP	Inferior hypogastric plexus
L&S	Latzko and Schiffmann
LP	Lateral parametrium
LUL	Lateral umbilical ligament
NSRH	Nerve-sparing radical hysterectomy
P&A	Peham-Americh
PSN	Pelvic splanchnic nerve
Q&M	Querleu and Morrow
RH	Radical hysterectomy
TA	Terminologia Anatomica
TCL	Transverse cervical ligament
TMMR	Total mesometrial resection
VUL	Vesicouterine ligament

1 Radical Hysterectomy in the Twentieth Century

The majority of radial hysterectomy (RH) carried out in the latter half of the twentieth century can be divided into two procedures: (a) non–nerve-sparing RH accompanied with excision of the lateral rectal ligament, a procedure, which was inherited from the L&S and Okabayashi procedures (Latzko and Schiffmann 1919; Okabayashi 1952a) and (b) nerve-sparing RH (Hoshiba et al. 2000; Yabuki et al. 2005; Yabuki 2019), accompanied with non-excision of the lateral rectal ligament advocated by the author. From a viewpoint of QOL, the L&S and Okabayashi procedures are provisionally designated as a conventional RH. The anatomy proposed by Savage/Kocks and Mackenrodt in the nineteenth century is referred to as classical anatomy (Mackenrodt 1895; Speert 1996; Savage 1870). Furthermore, Höckel's

The original version of the chapter has been revised. A correction to this chapter can be found at https://doi.org/10.1007/978-981-96-7194-6_5

Y. Yabuki, *Nerve-Sparing Radical Hysterectomy*,
https://doi.org/10.1007/978-981-96-7194-6_2

TMMR (2003) cannot be considered as a subject for discussion in the context of RH, for it is viewed as a modified Wertheim procedure, or semi-RH.

The characteristics of twentieth century RH are as follows: (a) inheritance of nineteenth century anatomy (Mackenrodt 1895; Savage 1870; Kocks 1880); (b) pursuit of extensive surgery for a radical cure (Latzko and Schiffmann 1919; Okabayashi 1921, 1952a; Meigs 1954); and (c) regarding new surgical procedures based on new surgical anatomy, nothing was published until the 1990s (Yabuki et al. 1991, 2000; Yabuki 1997) though radiotherapy and chemotherapy had developed.

In this chapter, L&S and Okabayashi's RH will be discussed and has been divided into the following: (1) parametrium/parametrectomy; and (2) paracolpium/paracolpectomy together with the author's views and recommendations.

2 Parametrium and Parametrectomy

2.1 Contradictions in Classical Parametrium

The author's study on the background of RH focused on two subjects: Latzko's surgical procedure from the English translation of "Operative Gynecology" by Peham-Amreich (P&A) published in 1934, and Hidekazu Okabayashi's Radical Operation for Carcinoma of the Uterine Cervix, or Systematic Radical Hysterectomy (Okabayashi 1921, 1952a), published in 1952.

Figure 2.1 demonstrates P&A's dense pelvic connective tissue that can be interpreted as being uniquely named by P&A. They also classified the lateral ligaments (i.e., pelvic connective tissue ground bundles) of the pelvic visceral organs into three categories: the horizontal connective tissue ground bundle, transitional zone, and frontal connective tissue ground bundle, with the pelvic visceral peritoneum serving as the boundary. The transitional zone is depicted merely as a blank space. Furthermore, they stated that the horizontal and frontal connective tissue ground bundles are almost perpendicular to each other, with the transitional zone in between. In the figure, the lateral ligament (pillar) of each organ is depicted as attaching parallel to the lateral aspects of their respective organ, as seen here represented by the lateral ligaments of the uterus and vagina. However, upon closer inspection of the diagram, the frontal connective tissue ground bundle is labeled as the Mackenrodt ligament, and its pelvic attachment is depicted as vertically arranged in three layers, rather than in a horizontal arrangement. In the English manual of P&A, the "connective tissue ground bundle" is translated from the original German term "Bindegewebsgrundstock," which is interpreted in the book as "Fascia endopelvina." From the German text, "Pfeiler" is translated into English as "pillar" or "septum" (Netter 2006).

However, the problematic point in Fig. 2.1 is that the frontal connective tissue ground bundle has been termed the Mackenrodt ligament. Mackenrodt himself referred to this lateral ligamentous structure of the cervix as the transverse or lateral cervical ligament. The term "Mackenrodt ligament" was coined later.

The author hypothesizes that P&A identified the frontal connective tissue ground bundle as the Mackenrodt ligament for the following reason: They likely adhered to

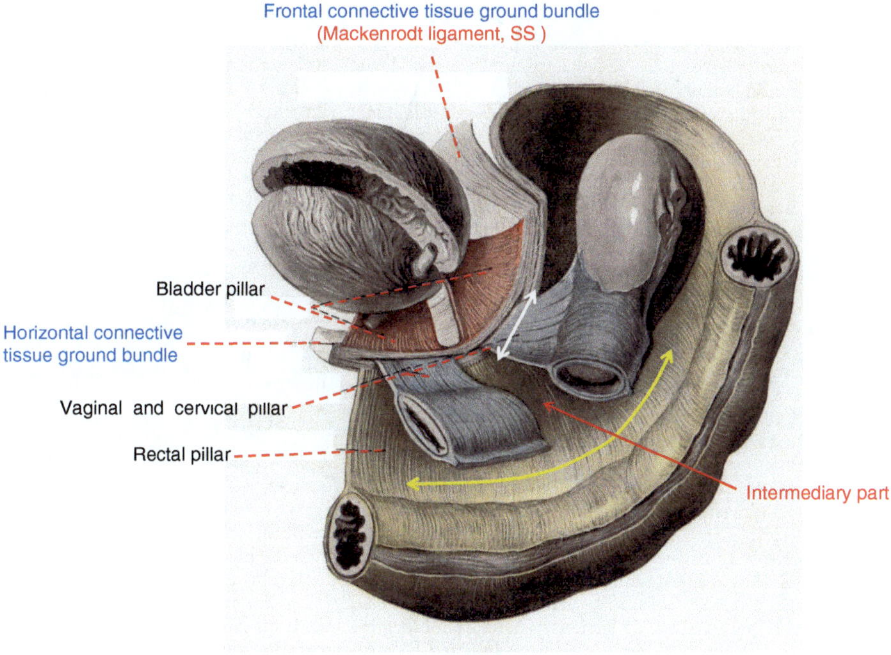

Fig. 2.1 Peham-Amreich's dense pelvic connective tissue
Each lateral ligament of the bladder, internal genitalia, and rectum is classified into the frontal connective tissue ground bundle, intermediary part, and horizontal connective tissue ground bundle. The ground bundles originating in the pelvic sidewall, called pillars, attach parallel to the lateral aspect of each organ. The intermediary part is considered relatively insignificant (red arrow). (Reproduced from Peham and Amreich 1930, Fig. 131, p.190)

Table 2.1 Classification by Peham and Amreich of dense connective tissue

	Pelvic connective tissue ground bundle	
	Frontal connective tissue ground bundle	Horizontal connective tissue ground bundle
Bladder pillar	Sagittal bladder pillar	Ascending bladder pillar
Vaginal-cervical pillar	Cervical pillar	Vaginal pillar
Rectal pillar	Sagittal rectal pillar	Descending rectal pillar

basic anatomical principles when considering the attachment site to the organs but relied on surgical observations when depicting the attachment to the pelvic wall, consequently blending both perspectives. At that time, surgical techniques and anatomical understanding had not sufficiently advanced to clearly distinguish between the two. The reason why the author focuses on P&A's surgical text is precisely because their contradictions provided valuable insights for further investigation. Furthermore, the vesicouterine and uterosacral ligaments are omitted from this figure.

Table 2.1 summarizes the pelvic connective tissue ground bundles as described by P&A. It is challenging in interpreting these terms to correspond to present-day terms for the ligaments.

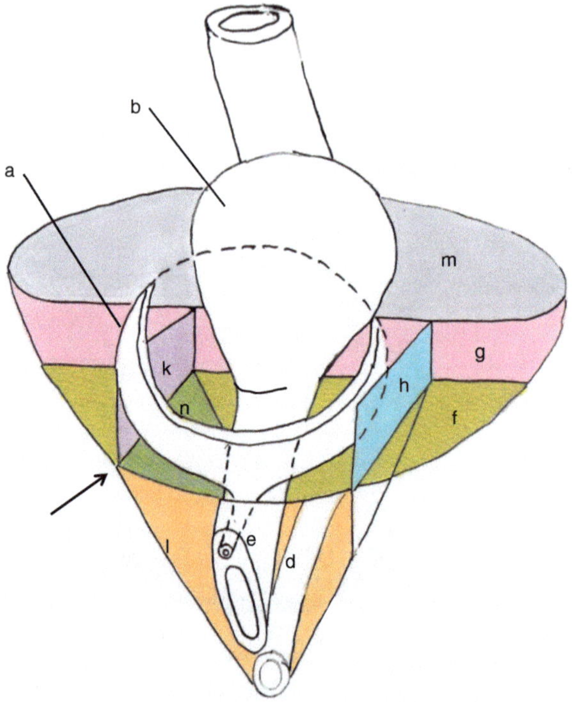

Fig. 2.2 Schematic representation of the pelvic connective tissue according to Amreich. (Adapted with permission from Reiffenstuhl 1982. ©Wolters Kluwer)
Taken from an article by Reiffenstuhl, this is a schematic illustration from Amreich's perspective, which has been colored and replicated by the author. Compared with Fig. 2.1 of P&A's illustration, Fig. 2.2 is of a more three-dimensional perspective as well as line diagrammatic in nature. However, it is difficult to discern the differences among ascending bladder pillar (**j**), sagittal bladder pillar (**k**), and bladder pillar (vesico-uterine ligament) (**h**). Furthermore, the frontal connective tissue ground bundle (**g**) appears synonymous with the cervical pillar and the horizontal connective tissue ground bundle (**f**) appears synonymous with the vaginal pillar
(**a**) urinary bladder, (**b**) uterus, (**d**) rectum, (**e**) vagina, (**f**) horizontal connective tissue ground bundle, (**g**) frontal connective tissue ground bundle, (**h**)bladder pillar (vesico-uterine ligament), (**j**) ascending bladder pillar, (**k**) sagittal bladder pillar, (**l**) descending rectal pillar, (**m**) sagittal rectal pillar, and (**n**) vaginal pillar

Figure 2.2 is a colored replica of Reiffenstuhl's 1982 illustration of Amreich's perspective. Reiffenstuhl, like P&A, classified the lateral supporter of the genital organs into frontal and horizontal connective tissue ground bundles but did not depict the intermediate zone. Although this is not clearly depicted in the figure, both ground bundles are described as being at a right angle at the junction of the uterus and vagina.

Reiffenstuhl's illustration, like P&A's, is also challenging to decipher. In his illustration, the frontal connective tissue ground bundle can be interpreted as the cervical pillar and is also referred to as the Mackenrodt ligament. Similarly, the horizontal connective tissue ground bundle can be identified as the vaginal pillar.

Reiffenstuhl's diagram is labeled as a "schematic representation of the pelvic connective tissue according to Amreich." Therefore, this should not be attributed as a misunderstanding by Reiffenstuhl, but rather considered an acknowledgment of the inconsistency in P&A's contradictions. Furthermore, there is still no explanation for the lateral rectal ligament.

P&A's Fig. 2.1 contains numerous difficult-to-interpret elements; however, the author attempted interpretations of panel (**a**) of Fig. 2.3 and Table 2.1. The terms in Table 2.1 were redefined as follows:

Sagittal bladder pillar ≑ vesicohypogastric fascia + anterior mesoureter
Cervical pillar = transverse cervical ligament
Sagittal rectal pillar ≑ lateral rectal ligament + posterior mesoureter
Ascending bladder pillar ≑ paracystium
vaginal pillar = paracolpium
Descending rectal pillar ≑ paraproctium

Readers are directed to refer to Figs. 3.30 and 3.31 for further details. However, these interpretations may be disputable.

According to Table 2.1, panel (**a**) of Fig. 2.3 divides P&A's lateral ligaments of the bladder, genital organs, and rectum into six pillars. Each pillar is independent, attaching parallel to the lateral aspect of the organs. The transitional zone and organs are depicted as blank spaces. Figure 3.4 is a depiction by the author of P&A's cross section in Fig. 2.1. In reference to P&A's Figs. 2.1 and 3.4, Netter (2006) created an illustration, titled "endopelvic fascia and potential spaces." It depicts potential

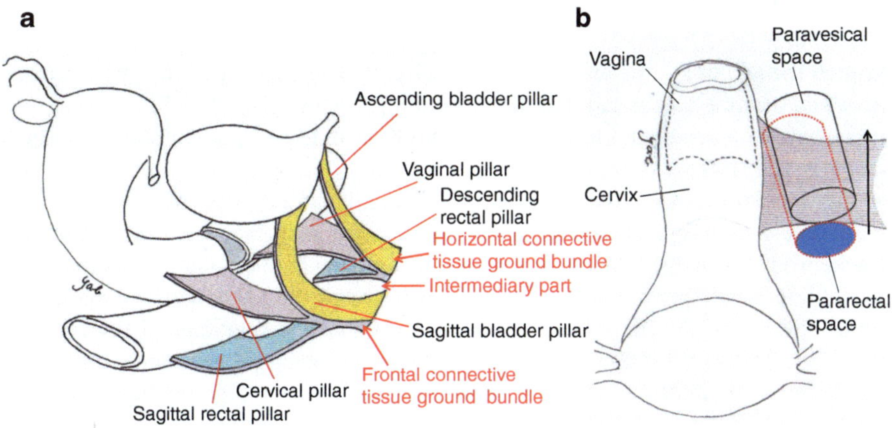

Fig. 2.3 Author's interpretation of P&A
Panel (**a**) is the author's interpretation of Fig. 2.1. Each lateral ligament of the pelvic organs is interpreted as an independent, horizontal, plate-like bundle connecting the lateral aspects of the pelvic sidewall. P&A's figure shows no indication of blood vessels
From a surgical perspective, panel (**b**) is a simplified schematic illustration based on Fig. 2.1. The paravesical and pararectal spaces are excavated along the ventral and dorsal aspects of TCL. Theoretically, the lateral parametrium, i.e., TCL, can be easily detached at the pelvic sidewall indicated by the black arrow

spaces parallel to the ventral and dorsal aspects of the parametrium, namely, the paravesical and pararectal spaces.

Panel (**b**) of Fig. 2.3 is a simplified surgical schematic illustration created by the author based on P&A and Netter's concepts. The author believes that apparent contradictions have persisted into the twenty-first century with P&A's era of confusion between the anatomy and surgical findings remaining partially unresolved. The author's intention was to solve these contradictions and establish a new theory and procedure.

Referenced from P&A's figures, dissection on fixed Japanese female cadavers was conducted by the author in the year 2000. Following opening of the abdominal cavity, the bladder and uterus/vagina were relatively easily dissected and separated. By severing the vesicouterine ligament and extending the gap laterally, the lateral ligament of the bladder was detached and, following dissection of the rectouterine/vaginal ligament, a similar procedure was carried out between the uterus/vagina and rectum, resulting in the separation of TCL. However, there was difficulty in distinguishing the lateral ligament of the rectum from the superior fascia of the pelvic diaphragm. Through this procedure, similar results were obtained to those depicted in P&A's figures. However, in actual surgery, the paravesical and pararectal spaces are excavated in a direction perpendicular to the organs. It can be concluded that a flaw of RH in the twentieth century lay in surgeons' unified approach to the anatomy and surgery based on the achievements of P&A and Reiffenstuhl.

2.2 *The Author's Perspective on the Conventional Parametrium*

Around the age of 50, the author, who had already had vast experience with numerous RHs, became convinced that the morphology of the dissected TCL, or cervical pillar, based on basic anatomy differed from that of TCL separated during surgery (Yabuki et al. 1991).

Panel (**a**) of Fig. 2.4, taken from P&A's surgical manual, appears to depict where the paravesical and pararectal spaces are perpendicularly excavated to separate the Mackenrodt ligament. In contrast, panel (**b**) depicts where the lateral parametrium, resembling a bat spreading its wings, is excised parallel to the lateral edge of the uterus (P&A 1934). These two figures suggest that the relationship between the uterus and Mackenrodt ligament fluctuates between being perpendicular and parallel. However, no matter how much the uterus is pulled cranially, the ligament separated between the two spaces cannot be considered horizontal to the uterus as depicted in panel (**b**) of Fig. 2.4. This is because, when the excised TCL, paracolpium and uterus/vagina are laid out on a board, they now appear two dimensional (Fig. 2.5) compared with appearing three dimensional during surgery.

Contradictions noted in Fig. 2.4 correspond to the questions the author came up with between cadaver dissection and then carrying out an actual surgical procedure. However, even today, it is common to encounter surgical manuals and articles that depict the morphology of TCL, which is similar to the observations expressed in

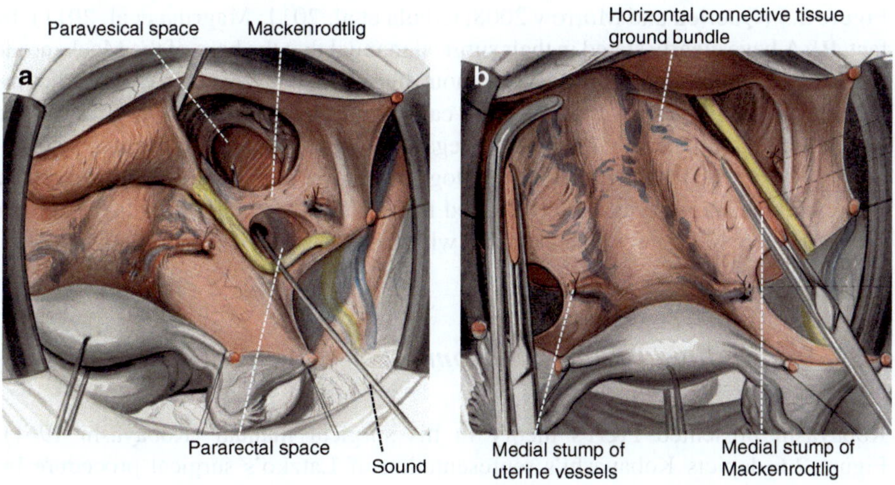

Fig. 2.4 Separation and severance of transverse cervical ligament in the Latzko procedure
Panel (**a**) depicts the excavated paravesical and pararectal spaces, thereby separating TCL. From the direction of the uterine sound insertion, the relationship between the uterus and TCL is presumably perpendicular. Also, the levator ani muscle is seen exposed
Panel (**b**) depicts the attachment of the Mackenrodt ligament and paracolpium parallel to the lateral aspect of the uterus and vagina. There is a large difference in illustration of the Mackenrodt ligament between panels (**a**) and (**b**) with panel (**a**) giving the impression of the Mackenrodt ligament being perpendicular and panel (**b**) of it being horizontal. (Reproduced from P&A 1930, Fig. 207 unt 213, p. 364 unt 372)

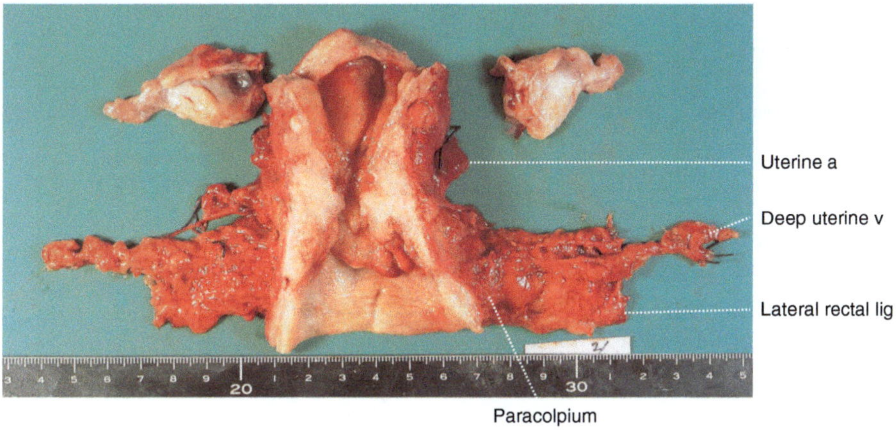

Fig. 2.5 Excised tissues from Okabayashi procedure
When the excised tissues, which were obtained from the author's procedure, are placed on a wooden board, one can see that the relationship between the uterus/vagina and the lateral ligaments loses its three-dimensional appearance and appears two-dimensional. Part of the tissue underneath the lateral ligament is the lateral rectal ligament

Figure 2.5 (Querleu and Morrow 2008; Cibula et al. 2011; Magrina et al. 2011). In fact, P&A have clearly stated in their surgical manual that the base of the Mackenrodt ligament is separated from the sacrospinous ligament, thereby clearly contradicting their own depictions seen in panel (**b**). It can be inferred that in the 1930s, it was not within the realm of acceptable practice regarding basic anatomy to assign new independent concepts, or terms, to morphology altered by artificial manipulation in a living body. Therefore, it can be inferred that the intraoperative findings shown in panel (**a**) were ultimately made to align with those in panel (**b**).

2.3 Conventional Parametrectomy

Kobayashi presented P&A's theory in his surgical manual (Kobayashi 1961). Figure 2.6 depicts Kobayashi's representation of Latzko's surgical procedure by P&A, which illustrates the relationship between the lateral parametrium, or Mackenrodt ligament, and pararectal space.

Kobayashi's diagram illustrates the pararectal space running alongside the rectum, but no precise location is specified, and it is partitioned craniocaudally by a septum (P&A explicitly identified this as the Mackenrodt ligament). P&A and Kobayashi referred to each partition as the "cephalic chamber" or upper portion of

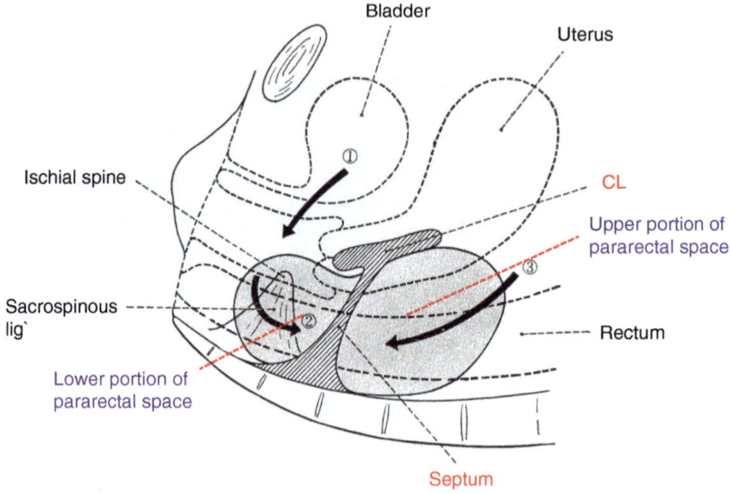

Fig. 2.6 Kobayashi's interpretation of the dense connective tissue of P&A
Seen here is the septum, which is referred to as the Mackenrodt ligament by P&A, separated between the lower and upper portions of the pararectal space and depicted as a bundle connecting CL, which is horizontal to the uterine cervix, and sacrospinous ligament. ①, ②, and ③ in this figure show the routes to the following: ① vesicouterine space; ② lower portion of the pararectal space; and ③ the upper portion of the pararectal space. (Reproduced from Kobayashi 1961, Fig. 84, p. 170, in Japanese)

the pararectal space and the "caudal chamber" or lower portion of the pararectal space, respectively (Fig. 2.6). Kobayashi's diagram excellently represents P&A's perspective. However, as seen in this figure, Kobayashi separately depicted CL parallel to the uterine axis and the septum supporting it from the sacrum but made no reference to this septum as the Mackenrodt ligament. Since the 1940s, Uhlenhuth et al. (1948) began using the term "cardinal ligament (of Mackenrodt)," and considered CL and TCL, or Mackenrodt ligament, as synonymous. Therefore, it is also likely why Kobayashi refrained from labeling the septum as the Mackenrodt ligament.

P&A described the creation of the two pararectal spaces in their surgical manual as follows (P&A 1934, p. 346): "If now a small sponge in a forceps is inserted downward against the loose connective tissue at the junction of the horizontal and frontal connective tissue ground bundles, an opening may be made into the lower portion of the pararectal space." Then P&A interconnected the two spaces as follows (P&A 1934, p. 346): "If the finger is then inserted from the upper portion of the pararectal space downward and forward to the pelvic floor, its tip will pass around the bend of the connective tissue ground bundle into the lower chamber of the combined pararectal and paravesical space. As the finger is passed from the cranial to the caudal chamber of the pararectal space it should pass along the sacrospinous ligament" (Fig. 2.7).

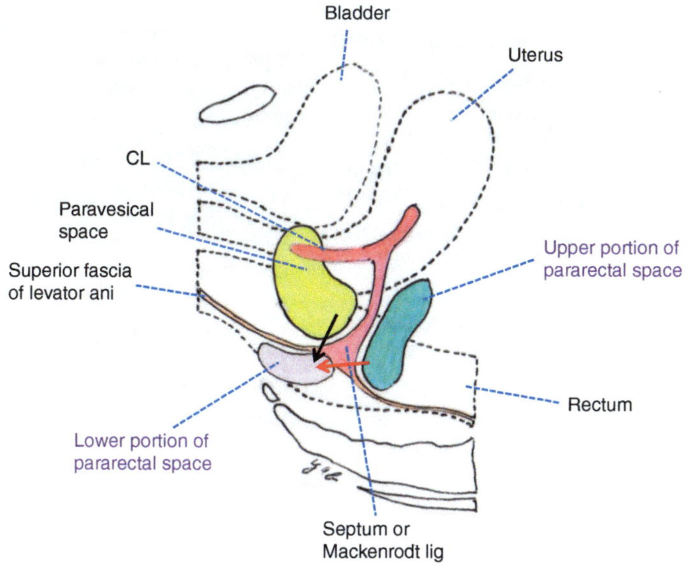

Fig. 2.7 Perpendicular paravesical space and upper/lower portions of the pararectal space
This is a faithful interpretation according to the description in P&A's surgical manual. First identified at the base of the paravesical space is the superior fascia of the levator ani muscle, and here the lower portion of the pararectal space is excavated (black arrow), and finally the base of the Mackenrodt ligament is breached through the upper portion of the pararectal space, creating a single pararectal space (red arrow)

Novice gynecologists attempting to visualize excision of the lateral parametrium will find P&A's two pararectal spaces a useful guide. However, in practice, it can be extremely challenging. Furthermore, the separation of the Mackenrodt ligament is described as follows in the figure legend of their surgical manual (Fig. 207 in P&A 1934, p. 347), and also in panel (**a**) of Fig. 2.3 in this book): "The tip of the sound may be seen in the paravesical space due to the fact that the posterior portion of the horizontal connective tissue ground bundle has been separated from the levator. The Mackenrodt ligament is therefore completely isolated."

The clamping of the Mackenrodt ligament in parametrectomy is shown by P&A (P&A 1934) in panel (**a**) of Fig. 2.8 and by Meigs (1954) in panel (**b**), respectively. Meigs stated that "The Web or ligament may appear to be rather thick, but, by careful picking, it may be cleaned of fatty tissue and thinned out so that it may be easily clamped along the pelvic wall." This figure clearly demonstrates the Mackenrodt ligament being clamped perpendicularly against the pelvic axis with forceps. However, in Meigs' surgery, there is no mention of excising the superior fascia of the levator ani, and the description is rather reminiscent of the Okabayashi procedure (Okabayashi 1921). This excision of the superior fascia of the levator ani may

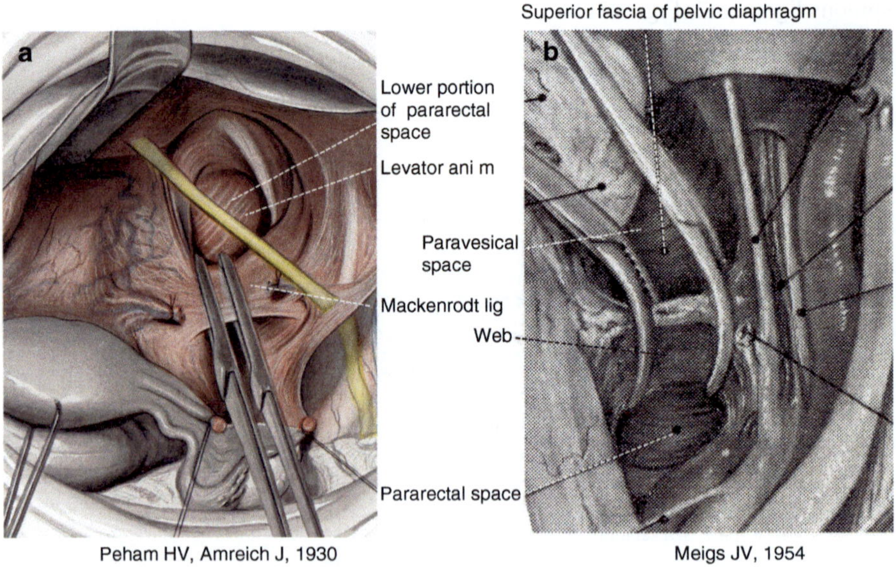

Fig. 2.8 Clamping of P&A and Meigs' Mackenrodt ligament
Although P&A and Meigs' excavation method for the spaces differs, they both clamp the Mackenrodt ligament perpendicularly and excise its base along the sacrospinous ligament. Meigs referred to the Mackenrodt ligament as the deep cardinal ligament or "Web" and wrote in his surgical manual, "After cutting the web, the floor of the pelvis becomes exposed." His method did not involve excising the superior fascia of the levator ani muscle and is rather similar to the Okabayashi procedure. (panel (**a**): Reproduced from P&A 1930, Fig. 208 , p. 364. Panel (**b**): Reproduced from Meigs 1954, Fig. 7, p. 175)

have served as a precursor to Höckel's (laterally) extended endopelvic resection (Höckel 1999).

2.4 The Author's Perspective on Conventional Parametrectomy

Panel (**a**) of Fig. 2.9 depicts the creation of the horizontal connective tissue ground bundle in a cadaveric model by the author and Murakami. When the superior fascia of the levator ani muscle is dissected from the levator ani muscle, the space created is the lower portion of the pararectal space. This superior fascia of the levator ani connects to the cross-sectioned lateral neurovascular bundles of the bladder, vagina, and rectum, becoming a mass on its medial aspect (Fig. 3.28).

P&A's panel (**b**) of Fig. 2.9 depicts the severed ends of the horizontal connective tissue ground bundle, the dissected rectal pillar along the rectum, and the stump of the Mackenrodt ligament. Unquestionably, this is consistent with the horizontal connective tissue ground bundle severed as indicated by the double-headed yellow arrow in Fig. 2.1. The reason for the excision of the rectal pillar in panel (**a**) of

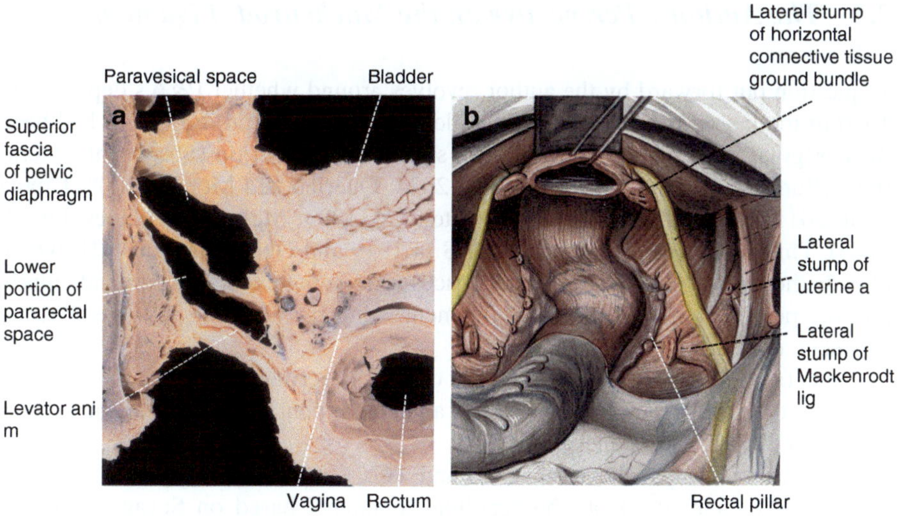

Fig. 2.9 Creation of and reasoning for the lower portion of the pararectal space
Panel (**a**) represents an image obtained by excising the paravesical space, superior fascia of the pelvic diaphragm, lower portion of the pararectal space, and levator ani muscle at the upper end of the vagina. (Reproduced from Yabuki et al. 2011)
The figure replicated in panel (**b**) is from Fig. 215 in P&A's surgical manual p. 356 and, the following is a quote taken from this manual concerning this figure: "On both sides of the rectum, almost the entire upper surface of the levator is exposed from the symphysis pubis to the sacrospinous ligament." The severed stump beside the rectum is considered to be the sagittal rectal pillar. However, panels (**a**) and (**b**) apply only to the horizontal connective tissue ground bundle that forms the lower portion of the pararectal space

Fig. 2.9 is that, when the superior fascia of the levator ani muscle is dissected on the parietal aspect, the neurovascular bundle on the visceral aspect of the bladder, vagina, and rectum remains a mass. As a result, to preserve the rectum, the rectal pillar must be once more resected at the side of the rectum illustrated in panel (**b**) of Fig. 2.9 (theoretically illustrated in Fig. 2.22). The same procedure applies to the bladder. This indicates that the excision of the horizontal connective tissue ground bundle was carried out in parallel. However, panel (**b**) of Fig. 2.8 shows that the Mackenrodt ligament was clamped perpendicularly relative to the uterine cervix and rectum. This indicates that the relationship between the cervical pillar, or TCL, and uterus is perpendicular, while that between the vaginal pillar and vagina is horizontal. P&A's unified approach for the cervical pillar, or TCL, and vaginal pillar may be explained by the following: (1) Their surgical technique is based on basic anatomic theory and (2) carrying out a more extensive and radical surgery compared to that of the Latzko/Okabayashi procedure.

It is indeed necessary to reexamine the relationship between the bladder and rectal pillars of the frontal and horizontal connective tissue ground bundles and their respective organs.

2.5 The Author's Perspective on the Mackenrodt Ligament

A question put forward by the author revolves around whether P&A's depiction in 1930 of the lateral parametrium as parallel to the uterus seen in Fig. 2.1 had been their original idea, and which has left a significant impact on subsequent generations (Ramirez et al. 2018; Plante et al. 2024; Querleu and Morrow 2008; Cibula et al. 2011; Magrina et al. 2011; Averette et al. 1993; Meigs 1945; Höckel et al. 2003). This is evident in surgery by L&S in 1919 and Okabayashi in 1921, where already the paravesical and pararectal spaces were being excavated perpendicularly and the perpendicular Mackenrodt ligament, or TCL including the lateral rectal ligament, excised.

Panel (**a**) of Fig. 2.10 is an illustration of TCL described in Mackenrodt's article (Mackenrodt 1895) in 1895. Panel (**b**) is an enlargement of the dashed square portion (detail window) in panel (**a**).

The author firmly believes that CL and TCL should be clearly distinguished. Kocks (1880) named CL as the "cardinal ligament" based on Savage's concept (Savage 1870), or the condensation in the base of the broad ligament. In articles on surgical procedures by Clark (1895) in 1895 and Wertheim (1912) in 1911, CL was defined and recognized as a bundle on the medial aspect of the ureter (Fig. 2.11).

The author had, at one time, simply considered Mackenrodt's TCL to be a plate-like extension of CL reaching to the pelvic wall (panel (**a**) of Fig. 2.3). However, Mackenrodt originally depicted it as a notch, or hole, shown in Fig. 2.10 where the uterosacral ligament attaches. Though it was unnamed at that time, from today's perspective, it is clearly the pararectal space. The following speculation by the

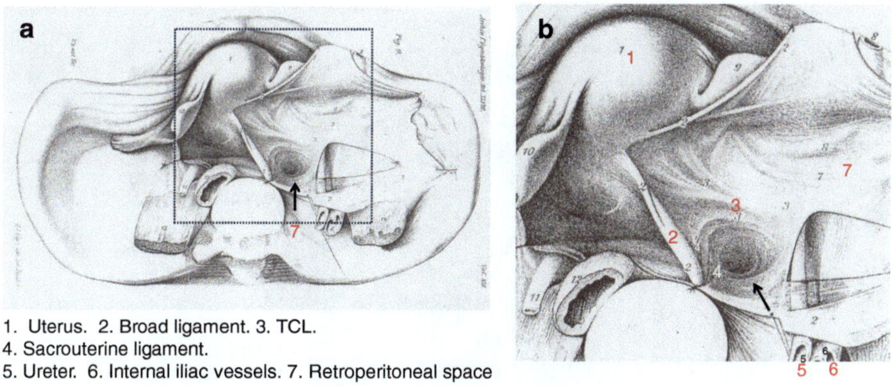

Fig. 2.10 The transverse cervical ligament of Mackenrodt
Viewed posteriorly, panel (**a**) is taken from an article by Mackenrodt, which depicts the uterus and right Mackenrodt ligament. A portion of the serosa of the uterine broad ligament is seen rolled superiorly, exposing TCL that connects the uterine cervix and pelvic sidewall. Here, the space that we now refer to as the pararectal space (black arrow) can already be observed. (Reproduced from Mackenrodt 1895, Fig. IX)
Panel (**b**) is an enlargement of the dashed square from the original diagram in panel (**a**). It can be inferred that Mackenrodt did not envision a board-like parametrium as depicted by P&A (panel (**a**) of Fig. 2.1), but rather a three-dimensional parametrium with the excavated space perpendicular to the lateral aspect of the uterosacral ligament

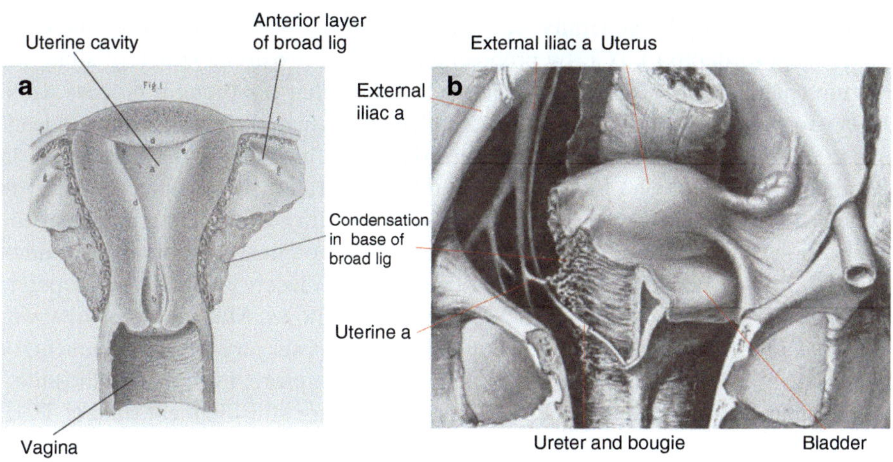

Fig. 2.11 The cardinal ligament of Savage/Kocks
Panel (**a**) is a diagram presented by Savage in 1870, illustrating the presence of pericervical tissue "the condensation in the base of the broad ligament" continuing from the uterine broad ligament. Kocks later named his concept of CL based on Savage's idea. (Reproduced from Savage 1880)
Panel (**b**) is a drawing taken from an article by Clark in 1985. A bougie is seen inserted into the ureter. CL is seen excised as a ligament on the medial aspect to the ureter, for, at that time, there was no concept of ligaments on its lateral aspect. Therefore, CL and TCL were not considered synonymous. (Reproduced from Clark 1895)

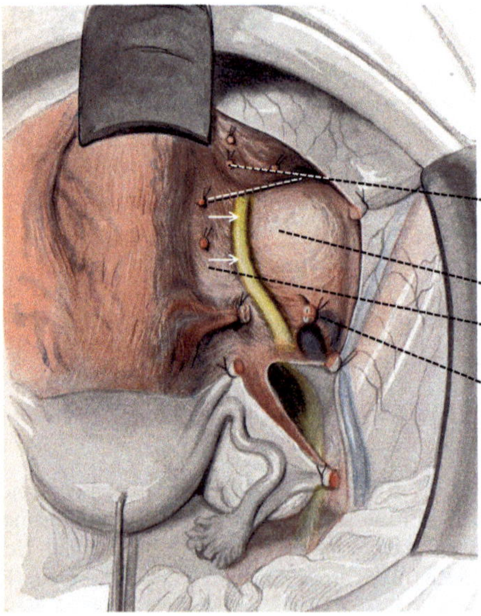

Fig. 2.12 Severance of the vesicouterine ligament in the Wertheim procedure
Seen are four stumps of the severed vesicouterine ligament, followed by severance of the uterine artery, exposing the anterior and middle portions of the ureter with lateralization. (Reproduced from P&A 1930, Fig. 205, p. 361)

author may already be generally well known of Mackenrodt having contributed to the concept of depth of TCL by proposing a three-dimensional structure along the sacrum (panel (**b**) of Fig. 2.10). It can be inferred that his thought process, from 1895 over a period of 20 years, conceptualized, progressed, and generalized, leading to eventual incorporation and application of it by L&S and Okabayashi. In Wertheim's article, "The Extended Abdominal Operation for Carcinoma Uteri in 1912," there is a passage as follows: "Mackenrodt criticizes us claiming that by the application of these clamps more parametrium is left on the pelvic floor. We cannot agree to this as happily, these clamps can be very closely applied on the pelvic floor." From this passage, the author speculates as follows: Mackenrodt's view was that the target for parametrium excision in Wertheim's surgery was the ligament, or CL, on the medial aspect of the ureter (Fig. 2.12). Therefore, even though the uterosacral ligament is resected at the pelvic floor, there are still ligament (lateral TCL) on the lateral aspect of the ureter that need to be excised.

There is no contradicting the fact that practical application of Mackenrodt's claim resulted in Latzko/Okabayashi's surgery. The Latzko/Okabayashi surgery is said to be a modification of the Wertheim procedure. However, the author believes that, without the introduction of Mackenrodt's theory, the two surgical procedures would not have similarly evolved. Wertheim's assertion of resecting the uterosacral ligament at the pelvic floor later followed with a view of seeking to categorize the

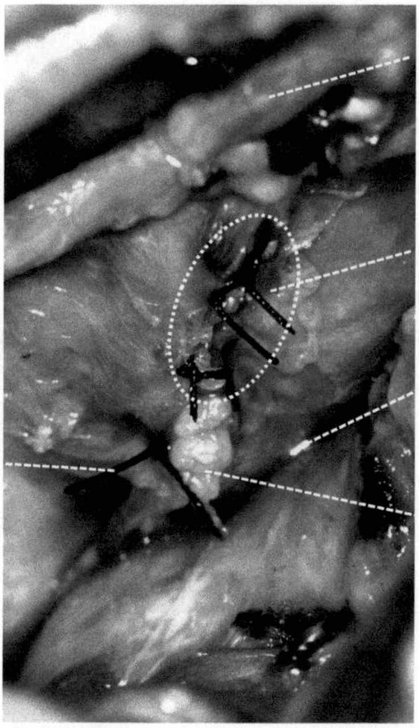

Fig. 2.13 Visceral branches' lateral stumps of the anterior trunks of the internal iliac vessels
An intraoperative photograph showing the separation of the vascular supporting system and its excision at the pelvic wall. The severed blood vessels are aligned in a single line perpendicular to the pelvic axis. This finding indicates that the relationship between SS and the pelvic organs becomes perpendicular during a surgical manipulation. (Reproduced from Yabuki et al. 1991)

Wertheim procedure as a type of RH (Ramirez et al. 2018; Plante et al. 2024) and also to claim that TCL and uterosacral ligament formed a common pedicle (Fig. 3.27) (Curtis et al. 1940).

Figure 2.13 is an intraoperative photograph of an RH carried out by the author in 1984. Based on many surgical manuals, the author believed at that time that the lateral parametrium existed horizontally and independently from the organs. To address the significant intraoperative hemorrhaging, the author separated and excised the blood vessels of the lateral parametrium one by one using CUSA, and then severed them at their origins (Yabuki et al. 1991). However, no matter how many times the blood vessels were severed, the arrangement of the disconnected vascular stumps appeared consistently perpendicular to the axis of the pelvis, rather than parallel. Moreover, Kobayashi (1961) stated that the lateral parametrium is composed of vascular and neural components in that order, but a pathology report of the author showed no nerve elements could be detected in the white stump seen on the lower part of Fig. 2.13. With the author's confusion peaking, he encountered Pernkopf's concept of the neurovascular stalk (Pernkopf 1943; Platzer 1989).

Figure 2.14 is a reproduction taken from Pernkopf's Topographische Anatomie des Menschen in 1943, Abb. 71.

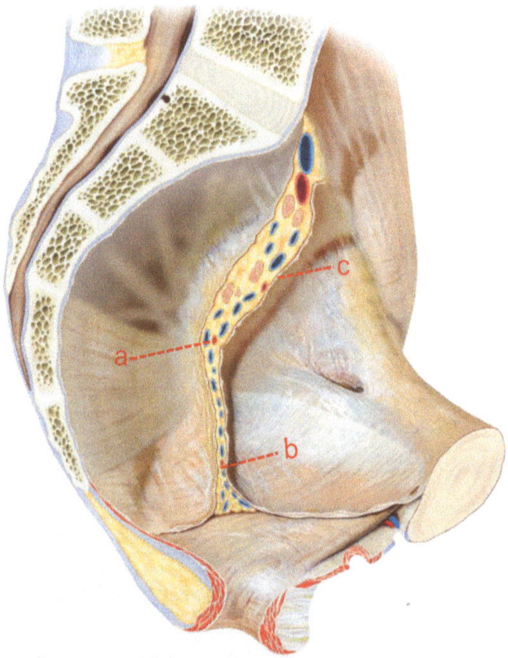

a) Inferior vesical a. b) Middle rectal a.
c) Visceral pelvic fascia.

Fig. 2.14 Pernkopf's neurovascular stalks of the pelvis
This diagram is reproduced from "Platzer W, ed. Pernkopf Anatomy, 3rd ed., Vol. II, Munich: Urban & Schwarzenberg, 1989, Fig. 286, p. 284," and the following is a quote from its figure legend: "View of left half. Midsagittal section through the male minor pelvis. Peritoneum and all organs are removed, and the parietal fascia is illustrated. The reflections of parietal fascia to visceral fascia, which invests individual organs, are seen. The neurovascular stalks run between the two fascial layers"

Figure 2.15 is a modification depicting a female by the author of the male figure from Pernkopf's Fig. 2.14. These two representations suggest that the lateral ligament of the bladder, uterus, and rectum does not form three separate plate-like structures like those depicted in panel (**a**) of Fig. 2.3, but rather constitute a continuum that is dorsoventrally, or perpendicularly, continuous.

A resemblance was also noted between Pernkopf's figure and the author's surgery (Fig. 2.13). Furthermore, in Fig. 2.14 of Pernkopf, the middle rectal artery is clearly indicated. Upon recognizing the presence of the lateral rectal ligament, the author became convinced that during RH, this ligament along with TCL can also be excised (Yabuki et al. 1991; Fig. 2.16).

Panel (**a**) of Fig. 2.17 depicts the gross anatomy and panel (**b**) a histological image of the pelvic organs, both of which were frontally sectioned through the vaginal part of the uterine cervix in a fixed cadaver. The organs are not precisely bisected in a symmetrical manner. As a result, on the left side of the rectangle in panel (**a**), the distribution of veins centered around the deep uterine vein can be identified. Panel (**b**) represents a histological cross section of the rectangle in panel (**a**), and TCL can be seen sandwiched between the area of two black dashed lines, including the stumps of the uterine artery and deep uterine vein. In addition, the region sandwiched between the two blue bold dashed lines represents the lateral rectal ligament and includes the middle rectal vessels penetrating the inferior hypogastric plexus. Also, in panel (**b**), the lesser pelvic cavity between the internal iliac vessels and vesicouterine vascular plexus (red double-headed arrow) is divided into two

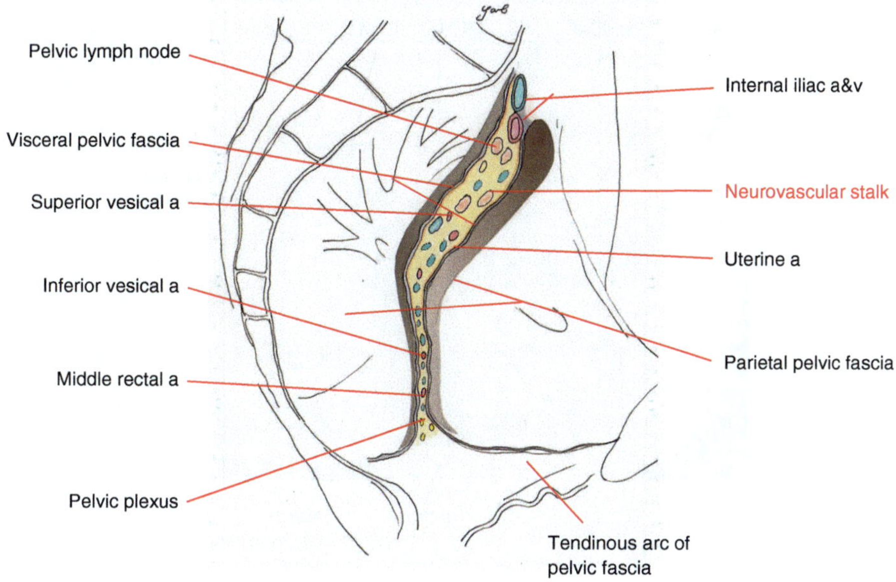

Fig. 2.15 Schematic illustration of the neurovascular stalks of the female pelvis
This illustration is drawn with reference to the neurovascular stalks of Pernkopf in the male pelvis cited in Fig. 2.14

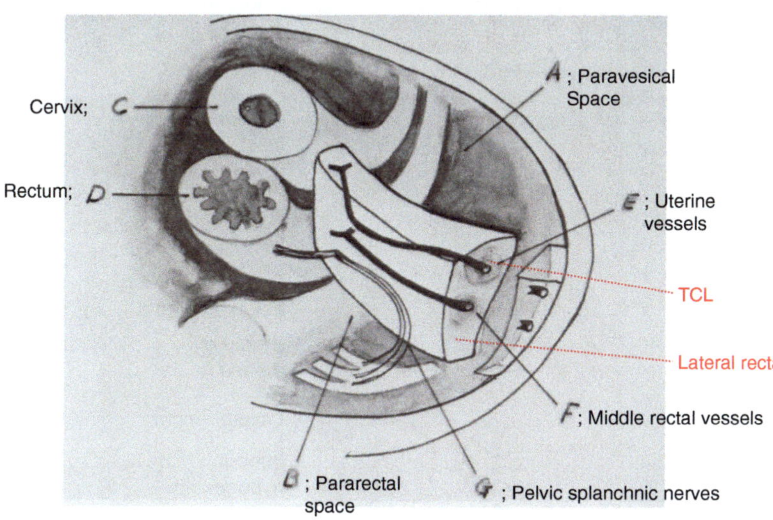

Fig. 2.16 Schematic illustration of the transverse cervical ligament and lateral rectal ligament
This illustration depicts TCL and lateral rectal ligament forming a continuum perpendicular to the organs. (Reproduced from Yabuki et al. 1991)

compartments by the inferior hypogastric plexus and vesical autonomic nerve branch extending from it. This nerve branches distributes to the bladder, and its pathway constitutes the posterior layer of Okabayashi's vesicouterine ligament

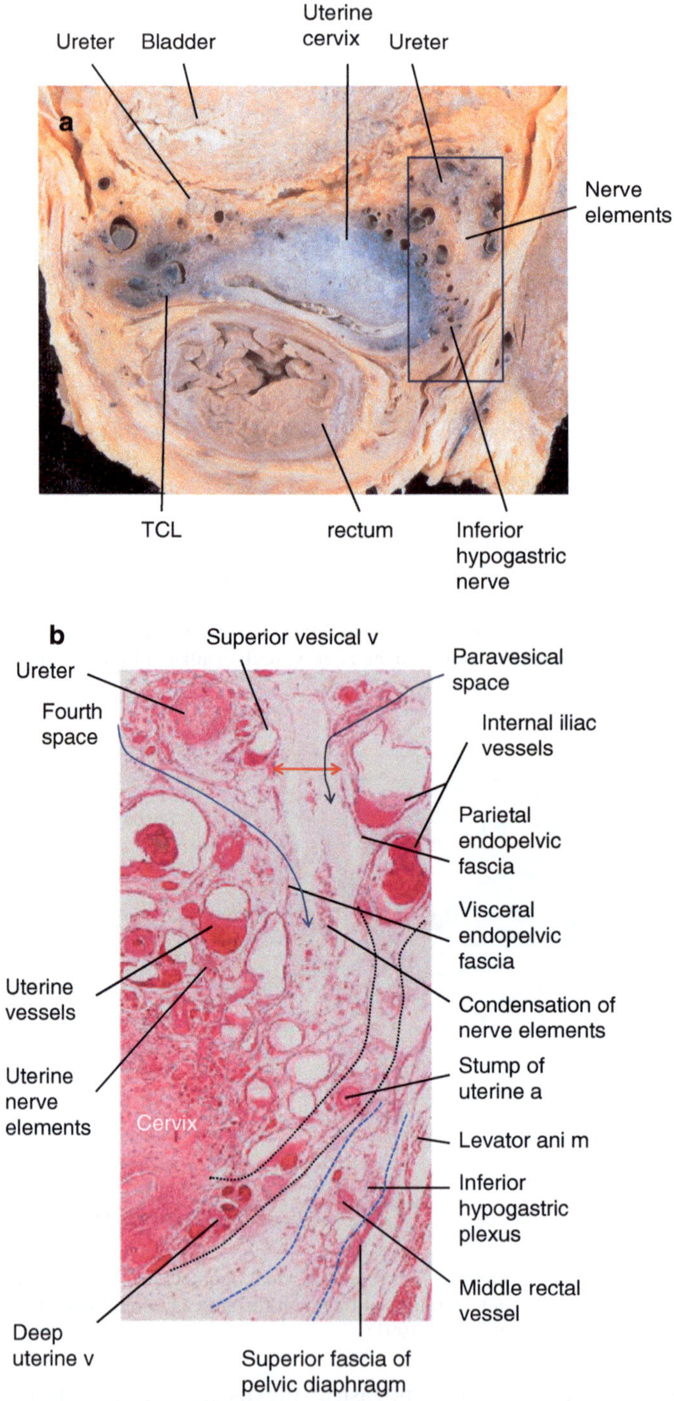
a
Ureter
Bladder
Uterine cervix
Ureter
Nerve elements
TCL
rectum
Inferior hypogastric nerve
b
Superior vesical v
Ureter
Fourth space
Paravesical space
Internal iliac vessels
Parietal endopelvic fascia
Visceral endopelvic fascia
Uterine vessels
Condensation of nerve elements
Uterine nerve elements
Cervix
Stump of uterine a
Levator ani m
Inferior hypogastric plexus
Middle rectal vessel
Deep uterine v
Superior fascia of pelvic diaphragm

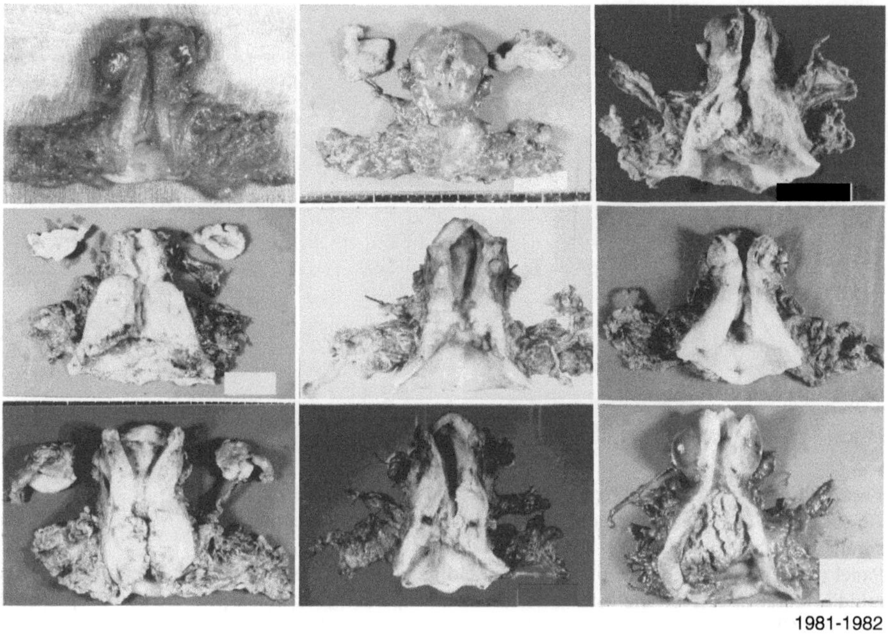

Fig. 2.18 Specimens extracted by the author following Okabayashi's radical hysterectomy procedure carried out from 1981 to 1982
Following excavation of the paravesical and pararectal spaces down to the pelvic floor, the parametrium, or TCL including the lateral rectal ligament, was revealed and then excised. Readers are asked to pay particular attention to the extensively excised parametrium

(Okabayashi 1952a). This tissue structure indicates that the lateral ligament of the bladder, uterus, and rectum forms a single dorsoventral plate, demonstrating that the relationship between the pelvic organs and lateral ligament is perpendicular.

Figure 2.18 shows specimens obtained from surgical procedures carried out by the author between 1981 and 1982, in which both the lateral rectal ligament and lateral parametrium have been simultaneously excised. Although endopelvic fascial resection was not carried out, the records show that each surgery resulted in more than 2000 ml of blood loss (Yabuki et al. 1991).

Fig. 2.17 Gross anatomy and histological image of frontally sectioned tissue through the vaginal part of the uterine cervix
Panel (**a**) shows severance from the anterior lip of the cervix to the upper end of the vaginal fornix in a slightly upward direction to the right. The autonomic nervous system appears to be interrupted by TCL. (Reproduced from Yabuki et al. 2011)
Panel (**b**) is an enlarged histological image corresponding to the black rectangle in panel (**a**). The nerve elements that extend linearly from the inferior hypogastric plexus to the bladder are the vesical autonomic nerve branches. The surrounding areas of the vesical nerve branches are filled with areolar connective tissue, forming two compartments, or the fourth and paravesical spaces, with the visceral endopelvic fascia on the medial aspect and parietal endopelvic fascia on the lateral aspect. (Reproduced from Yabuki 2023)

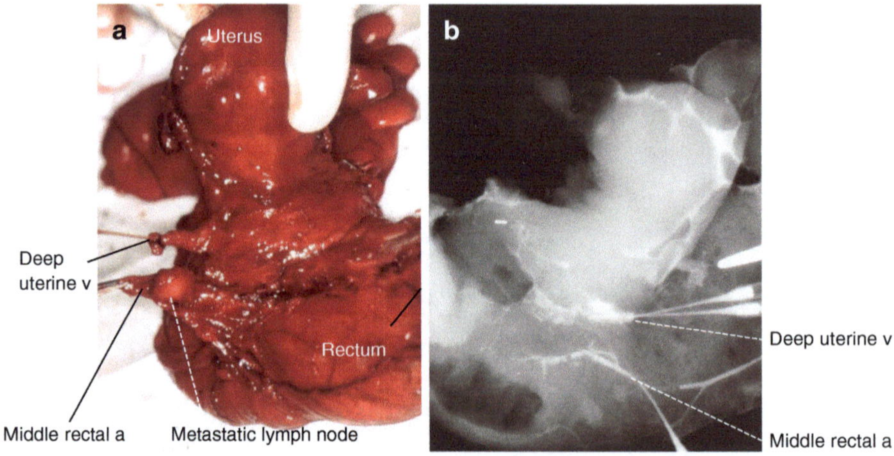

Fig. 2.19 Specimen excised by a combined rectal transection RH
An abdominoperineal resection and RH for advanced rectal cancer were carried out simultaneously
Panel (**a**) depicts a specimen of the uterus and rectum showing a metastatic lymph node of the middle rectal artery, or the lateral rectal ligament, on the dorsal aspect of the deep uterine vein, or TCL
Panel (**b**) shows the deep uterine vein and middle rectal artery injected with a contrast medium to enable visualization of the relationship between TCL and lateral rectal ligament. (Reproduced from Yabuki et al. 1991)

To further a greater understanding of the relationship between TCL and the lateral rectal ligament, the author actively participated in surgeries for rectal cancer. Furthermore, he combined RH with surgery for rectal cancer when infiltration into the lateral rectal ligament had occurred.

Panel (**a**) of Fig. 2.19 shows a specimen in which the lateral ligaments of both the rectum and uterus were simultaneously excised. By injecting contrast medium into the deep uterine vein and middle rectal artery of the specimen, it could be confirmed that TCL and the lateral rectal ligament, which appeared continuous during surgery, could be separated (panel (**b**)). During this time, the pathology reports of past specimens were reexamined and, as a result, no infiltration or metastasis of cervical cancer was detected in the tissues corresponding to the lateral rectal ligament.

2.6 The Author's Parametrectomy and Discussion

In 1985, based on past experiences, the author decided on and initiated a new approach to surgery for cervical cancer by carrying out excision of only TCL while preserving the lateral rectal ligament (Fig. 2.16). Using liposuction or CUSA (Rose et al. 1999), the author removed the fascia, the adipose tissue, and loose connective tissue covering TCL, and separated the blood vessels (Fig. 2.20). At the same time, the excavation of the paravesical and pararectal spaces was extended to the level of

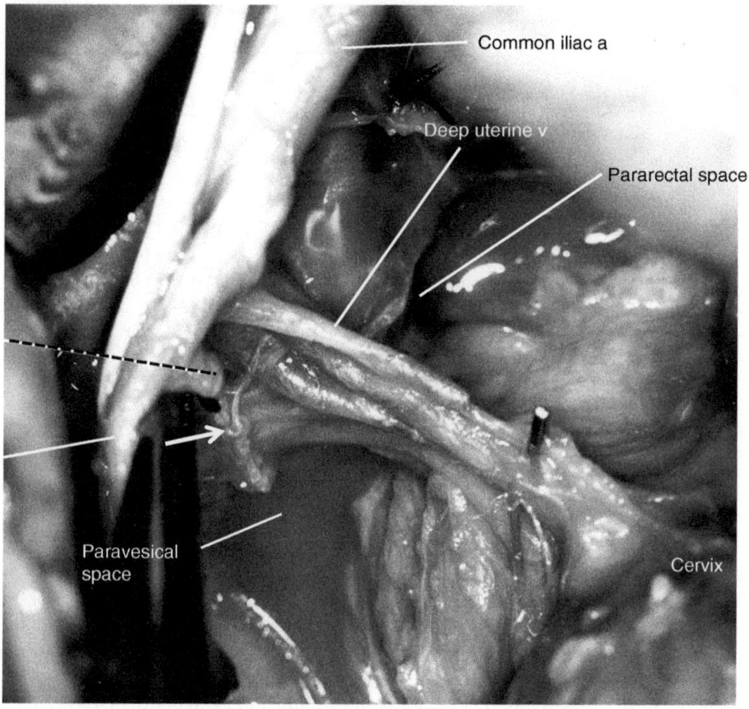

Fig. 2.20 Separation of the visceral branches from the anterior trunks of the internal iliac vessels An intraoperative photograph with the visceral fascia (white arrow) excised, exposing the visceral branches of the anterior trunks of the internal iliac vessels with the uterine artery already severed, and the deep uterine vein, inferior vesical vein, middle rectal vein, and coccygeus muscle dissected. The parametrium, or Mackenrodt ligament equivalent to TCL including the lateral rectal ligament, as seen excised as in Latzko/Okabayashi conventional RH suggests that these vessels were a bundle covered with fascia (white arrow). (Reproduced from Yabuki et al. 1991)

the uterus/vagina with only the vessels of TCL, or uterine artery, and/or superficial/deep uterine veins, being excised, while leaving the lateral rectal ligament intact.

This use of CUSA was combined with thorough irrigation and suction of the surgical field to minimize concerns regarding the dissemination of disrupted cancer cells (Yabuki et al. 1991; Oosterhuis et al. 1985). This manipulation led to a successful reduction in the amount of hemorrhage during parametrectomy (Fig. 2.21).

However, another issue still remained regarding crucial management of hemorrhage during the excision of the vesicouterine ligament (Fig. 2.21) (Rose et al. 1999). But, resolution of this issue had to wait some years until the discovery of the nerve-sparing procedure (Yabuki 1997; Yabuki et al. 2000). The aforementioned surgical findings were submitted and accepted for publication in the AJOG in 1991 (Yabuki et al. 1991). However, the reviewers did not address their perspective on the traditional resection of the lateral parametrium as a complex of TCL and the lateral rectal ligament. The author believes that the non-excision of the lateral rectal ligament was indeed a pivotal discovery regarding reduction in blood loss together with minimal invasive surgery. Furthermore, this manipulation was a stepping stone for

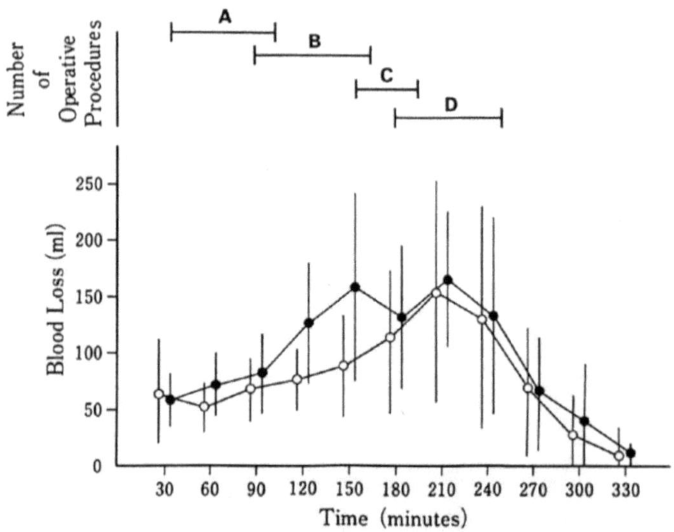

Fig. 2.21 The effect of non-excision of the lateral rectal ligament
Here follows a quote from the legend in the author's figure published in AJOG (1991). "Comparison of intraoperative bleeding measured at 30-min intervals, between standard RH (total volume, 1092±359 ml; operation time, 300±32 minutes) and RH by our method (total volume, 850±290ml; operation time, 296±36 min). In the latter case, blood loss measured at 120 and 150 min was 75±27 and 86±44 ml, respectively. These values are significantly smaller than the counterparts of (127±51 and 158±83 ml) for the former ($p<0.05$). (**a**) Dissection of intrapelvic lymph nodes; (**b**) dissection of CL; (**c**) severance of uterosacral and rectovaginal ligaments; (**d**) severance of vesicouterine ligament and paracolpium." (Reproduced from Yabuki et al. 1991)

the future nerve-sparing procedure. It has been established that when TCL and the lateral rectal ligament are simultaneously excised in conventional surgery, it is necessary to reexcise the lateral rectal ligament in the vicinity of the rectum to separate the uterus from the rectum (Fig. 2.22). This is clearly suggested in the excision of the rectal pillar shown in panel (**b**) of Fig. 2.9 by P&A.

Furthermore, excessive excavation of the pararectal space resulted in the connection of the left and right pararectal spaces on the posterior surface of the rectum (red curved arrows in Fig. 2.22). The hemorrhaging resulting from the ruptured venous plexus covering this exposed sacral surface was difficult to control, and the author's experience of it left an indelible effect.

In 1997, the author participated in a journal symposium on the parametrium and paracolpium organized by Morrow titled: "The parametrium and paracolpium: It was an anatomic and surgical symposium with emphasis on the cardinal ligament as it relates to radical hysterectomy" (Yabuki 1997). In the journal discussion, the author spoke on the conventional concept of the lateral parametrium, which includes the lateral rectal ligament, and implications concerning the effect of preservation surgeries. In addition, he elaborated on his nerve-sparing procedure introduced in 1996. During the same symposium, an article presented by Dr. T and colleagues included the following statement concerning the vein in CL: "The veins of the

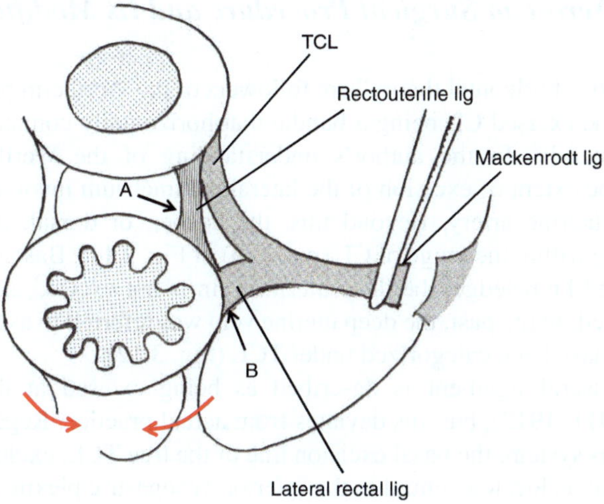

Fig. 2.22 A surgical contradiction in which the lateral rectal ligament is included in the parametrium
In conventional RH for total separation of the uterus and rectum, clamping with en bloc excision of the parametrium, or TCL including the lateral rectal ligament, requires not only severance of the uterosacral ligament (arrow A) but also re-excision of the rectal attachment of the lateral rectal ligament (arrow B). (Reproduced from Yabuki et al. 1991)

uterus collect at the lateral border of the uterus to form an impressive uterovaginal venous plexus that runs off through the cardinal ligament to the internal iliac vein at the pelvic side wall. Surgically, the cardinal ligament seems to consist more of veins than anything else." These observations by Dr. T and his colleagues suggest that, in the 1990s, the existence of the lateral rectal ligament may not have been fully recognized in gynecology. In response, the Editor's note stated: "See Yabuki for discussion of the uterine veins." Editor's conclusion was as follows: "Yoshihiko Yabuki presents a very detailed analysis of the structure of the parametrium, its relationship to the autonomic innervation of the pelvic organs and radical hysterectomy, and the sequelae of radical hysterectomy" (Yabuki 1997).

From the time of Latzko's publication in 1919 (Latzko and Schiffmann 1919) until 1991 (Yabuki et al. 1991) when the author stated it in an article (Querleu and Morrow 2008), he discovered that no one had acknowledged this intraoperative finding of the lateral rectal ligament, even though it was obviously visualized when extended surgery was most eagerly pursued. The reason for this may be due to the following issues: (a) a customary accepted rule among gynecologists that one must historically and traditionally not stray from basic anatomy and (b) the closed nature and/or factional character of gynecologist society. These reasons may have acted as a hindrance to solving the discrepancy between the theory of anatomy and practical application of it in surgery. One simpler explanation is that believers in P&A's horizontal theory of the parametrium have never doubted that the lateral rectal ligament as being a portion of the parametrium (Querleu and Morrow 2008; Cibula et al. 2011; Magrina et al. 2011; DeLancy 1992).

2.7 The Wertheim Surgical Procedure and Its Modifications

Believers of the "horizontal theory" are followers of the Wertheim procedure with a rationale of the excised CL being a bundle that horizontally connects to the ureter and uterine cervix. In the author's understanding of the Wertheim operation (Fig. 2.23), the extent of excision of the lateral parametrium involves isolating and excising the uterine artery. Beyond this, the deeper, or dorsal, area is resected approximately within the range of CL (panel (**b**) of Fig. 2.11). Based on the author's experience and knowledge, the deep uterine vein is not excised although it is not explicitly stated. In the past, the deep uterine vein was referred to as the vaginal vein and may not have been categorized under TCL (Fig. 3.12).

The uterosacral ligament is described as being excised at the pelvic floor (Wertheim 1911, 1912), but this deviates from actual practice. Regarding the autonomic nervous system, the basal excision line of the true TCL, excluding the lateral rectal ligament, is located ventral to the inferior hypogastric plexus, or dorsal to the deep uterine vein. In the Wertheim procedure in which the deep uterine vein is preserved, the autonomic nerves are inevitably preserved. In addition, this procedure does not incorporate Okabayashi's concept of the posterior layer of the vesicouterine ligament, and, as a result, the nervous system is neither exposed nor excised. One drawback perceived by the author in the Wertheim procedure is the concern that, due to the clamping, transection, and ligature of CL along with the fascia, the

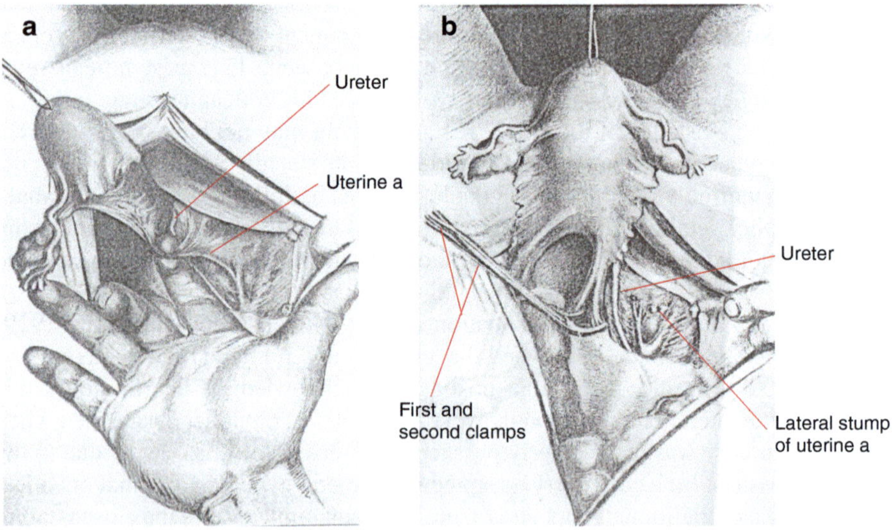

Fig. 2.23 Wertheim procedure
Panel (**a**): The index finger is seen inserted beneath the vessel bundle, lifting it away from the upper surface of the midureter. This vessel bundle including the uterine artery forms the roof of the ureteral canal in CL
Panel (**b**) shows the first clamping of the uterosacral ligament with Wertheim forceps and second clamping of CL. (Reproduced from Wertheim 1912)

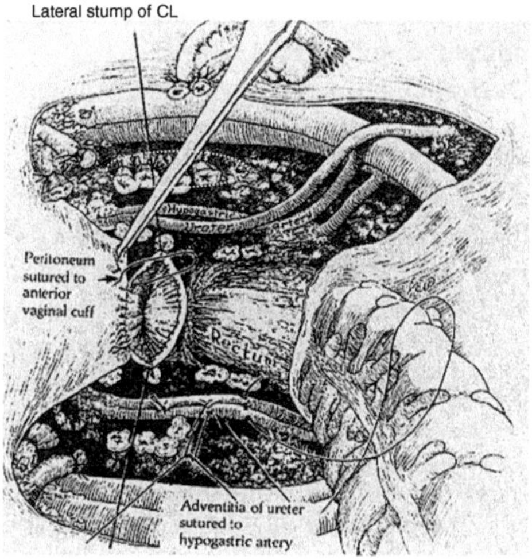

Fig. 2.24 Wertheim-Meigs radical hysterectomy advocated by Averette et al.
This is a surgical procedure adapted for stage IB–IIA. The Meigs procedure, which he presented in 1944, is believed to be a modified version of the Wertheim procedure. Certainly, the neatly aligned stumps of the excised parametrium along the axis of the pelvis are indicative of a Wertheim procedure (please compare with Fig. 2.13). The 5-year survival rate for this procedure was 90.1%

lymphatic drainage system may be trapped within the area of external ligation (Fig. 2.23).

In Fig. 2.24, Averette et al. (1993) illustrate what was known as a modified Wertheim RH. In this procedure, while introducing excavation of the paravesical and pararectal spaces and carrying out lymph node dissection, CL is divided into anterior and posterior portions and then excised. The author believes that this anterior portion corresponds to "unroofs" of the ureter (panel (**a**) of Fig. 2.23) in the Wertheim procedure and the posterior portion to Wertheim's CL excision by second forceps (panel (**b**)). However, the Averette procedure does not aim for excision of the deep uterine vein, and the author does not recognize this procedure as an RH. Naturally, in this modified Wertheim procedure, there is no mention of the lateral rectal ligament.

In an article on surgery for rectal cancer in 1908, the lateral rectal ligament was described in the field of gastrointestinal surgery by Miles (1908), and the 36th British edition of Gray's Anatomy quoted on this ligament in 1980: "The fascia around the middle rectal vessels passes from the posterolateral wall of the lesser pelvis (at the level of the third sacral vertebra) to the rectum, constituting on each side the lateral ligament of the rectum." However, there is no mention of its relation to the parametrium. Even among gastrointestinal surgeons in the 1980s, there was little interest in the lateral rectal ligament. One reason for this being that, in total mesorectal excision (TME), which is the standard surgery for rectal cancer, the middle rectal vessels are excised on the medial aspect of the inferior hypogastric plexus (Heald et al. 1982; Heald 1988; Enker et al. 1995; Moriya et al. 1989; Sugihara et al. 2006). As a result, the surgeon did not have the opportunity to separate and observe the lateral rectal ligament. Another reason is, in rectal cancer, hepatic metastasis frequently occurs through lymphatic drainage around the superior rectal vessels, so lateral dissection of the pelvis is considered to be insignificant (Sugihara et al. 2006).

Heald et al.'s TME is a novel concept based on embryologic development. The author has heard that Höckel et al.'s TMMR was based on ontogenetic anatomy inspired by Heald et al.'s TME (Heald et al. 1982; Heald 1988). Heald studied the morphogenesis of the hindgut and mesorectum, while Höckel that of the Müllerian duct and mesometrium, thereafter incorporating these developmental forms into their respective surgical techniques (Höckel et al. 2005, 2009; Höckel 2007).

The rectum originates from the endoderm hindgut of the embryonic foregut, while the mesorectum supports the terminal portion of the intestinal tract during fetal development. The author had the strong impression that, in adults, the extent of rectal resection took precedence over defining the mesorectum. In fact, in Heald's 1982 article (Heald et al. 1982), the tissues posterior to the rectum were excised as the mesorectum, but by 1998 (Heald 1988), the focus shifted to removing all tissues surrounding the rectum, with the introduction of the term "the holy plane." Höckel et al.'s surgical theory that focuses on the removal of the Müllerian anlage has shown excellent results when used for early-stage cancer of the uterine cervix. However, the reasons for not including the deep uterine vein in the resection area of the Müllerian unit have not been clearly elucidated.

Pelvic organs constitute an assembly with different functions, and the ontogenetic anatomy of the supporting structures surrounding these organs is of utmost interest to surgeons. In Höckel's surgical videos, it appears that he considers the lateral umbilical ligament/vesicohypogastric fascia as the bladder mesentery and surgically preserves it (Höckel 2007). This procedure is one that is routinely carried out in RH, so it cannot be considered a distinctive feature of TMMR. Höckel's excision of the bladder pillar, or the anterior layer of Okabayashi's vesicouterine ligament, is carried out in a similar manner to that of the Okabayashi procedure (Höckel 2007). However, in Höckel's approach, no manipulation is carried out on the posterior layer of Okabayashi's vesicouterine ligament. Is Höckel denying the existence of the neurovascular connection between the bladder and deep uterine vein? Or is he considering it as the bladder mesentery, and therefore not targeting it for excision? Also, his surgical technique does not address excision of the deep uterine vein. The deep uterine vein was previously referred to as the vaginal vein. It is a well-known fact that the deep uterine vein joins the internal iliac vein via the uterine cervix and TCL (Yabuki et al. 1991). The superior vesical vein within the Okabayashi's posterior layer drains into the deep uterine vein (Yabuki 1997). In fact, metastasis to the posterior layer of Okabayashi's ligament in cervical cancer is rare. There is an article by Kraima et al. titled "The vesicouterine ligament does not contain lymphatics from the uterine cervix" (Hoshiba et al. 2000). However, this should be considered separately from the fact that the posterior layer is bladder mesentery. Furthermore, the author does not believe that TMMR can always be applied to barrel-shaped 2FIGO IB3 or FIGO IIB cervical cancer, even when combined with neoadjuvant chemotherapy. Höckel considers the Wertheim procedure as a modification of the conventional abdominal RH and refers to his own surgery as a modified RH. The author is reminded of the discussion between Wertheim and Mackenrodt, as described on p. 26 and reasons why TMMR should not be classified within the scope of RH. He also believes that the primary reason for the excellent outcome of TMMR (Höckel et al. 2003) is Höckel's outstanding surgical skill combined with another contributing factor of his thorough lymphadenectomy achieved through the excavation of the paravesical and pararectal spaces. However, based on the author's experience, he questions the need, in early-stage cancer, to emphasize separation of the hypogastric nerve and/or extensive excision of the uterosacral ligament and the posterior leaf of the uterine broad ligament.

Although it may be trivial, the author finds himself unable to fully interpret in totality TME and/or TMMR. Heald's excision line is delineated along the visceral fascia and resected in an elliptical manner. In contrast, the original diagram by Enker (Enker et al. 1995) in 1992 depicts the lateral ligament and middle rectal artery within the lateral excision line of the mesorectum. There are doubts regarding whether Höckel completely excises TCL.

The author speculates that articles on twenty-first century RH by Magrina et al. (2011), Cibula et al. (2011), and Ramirez et al. (2018) also show a strong awareness of the Wertheim operation. Moreover, it has been reported in an article by Plante that, in low-risk cervical cancer, there was no difference in pelvic recurrence at 3 years in patients who underwent a simple hysterectomy or type II RH (Plante et al. 2024). The author does not agree with European Organisation for Research and Treatment of Cancer (EORTC) type II (Verleye et al. 2009), Piver class II (Piver et al. 1974), and Q&M type B (Querleu and Morrow 2008) operations being true RHs. Nevertheless, the article by Plante et al. (2024) suggests narrowing future surgery for cervical cancer down to simple hysterectomy and nerve-sparing RH. However, NSRH may very likely be replaced by CCRT in the future.

3 Parametrectomy by Peham-Amreich's Latzko Method and Okabayashi's Parametrectomy

The author who personally experienced the Okabayashi procedure (Okabayashi 1952a), which shifted toward over-resection, seriously felt the need to reexamine this procedure including that of L&S from a perspective of the basic and clinical anatomies. Nevertheless, despite the drawbacks, these pioneering surgical procedures left behind by L&S and Okabayashi are truly like precious jewel to gynecologists. However, it can be understood from P&A's Latzko procedure that even the surgical techniques of L&S and Okabayashi were still in the developmental stage. The author believes that, to enable modification of these imperfect aspects of the latter's surgery into surgical techniques suited for today's QOL, it is necessary to study and reevaluate their procedures rather than the Wertheim procedure. Even without actually having experienced the L&S and Okabayashi procedures, having had acquisition to their pioneering knowledge can lead to further advancement in understanding of pelvic anatomy and therefore deal with unexpected surgical incidents. These RH procedures of L&S and Okabayashi are to be described by dividing them into three manipulations: (1) anterior manipulation that is focused on the excision of the vesicouterine ligament, (2) posterior manipulation that is focused on the excision of the uterosacral/rectouterine ligaments, and (3) lateral manipulation that is focused on the excision of TCL.

3.1 Anterior Manipulation

3.1.1 The Okabayashi Procedure (Okabayashi 1952a)

In Okabayashi's anterior manipulation, the vesicouterine pouch is created, followed by the anterior and posterior layers of the vesicouterine ligament individually excised. By this procedure, the uterus/vagina is detached from the bladder essentially within the excision area (Fig. 2.25) with the lateral umbilical artery/ligament and vesicohypogastric fascia being preserved.

The concept of the vesicouterine ligament in the Okabayashi procedure represents an independent field of thought that could be termed as clinical anatomy being distinct from that of basic anatomy. That is to say, the vesicouterine ligament has been classified into the anterior and posterior layers, which are composed of a

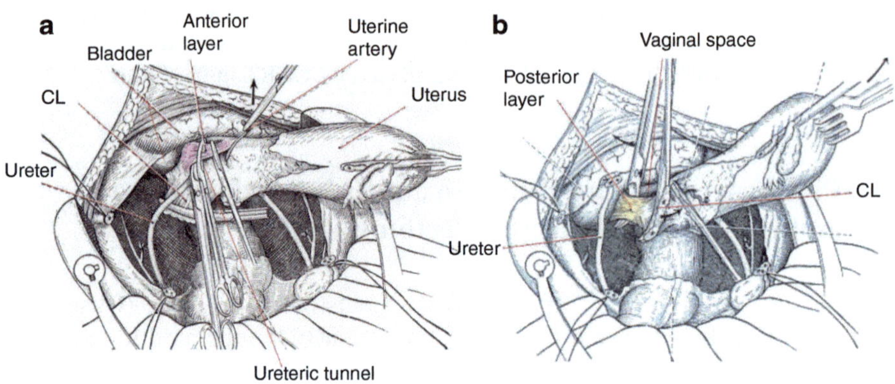

Fig. 2.25 Excision of Okabayashi's anterior and posterior layers of the vesicouterine ligament
Panel (**a**) depicts severance of the anterior leaf of the vesicouterine ligament. This is carried out by grasping the medial stump of the uterine artery with Pean forceps and then inserting Cooper scissors along the medial aspect of the ureter to excavate the ureteral tunnel. This is followed by severance of the anterior leaf of the vesicouterine ligament, or *ureteric roof*, between the two clamps, repeating this procedure two to three times to create the paravaginal space
Panel (**b**): This is a diagram reproduced from Okabayashi depicting severance of the posterior leaf of the vesicouterine ligament with a description: "illustrating the insertion of Cooper scissors into the paravaginal space, spreading them widely to free the posterior leaf of the vesicouterine ligament." The tip of the scissors can be seen protruding into the paravesical space. (Reproduced from Okabayashi 1952b, Fig. 26, p. 33, in Japanese)

different structure than that of the pubocervical ligament and bladder pillar. The anterior layer corresponds to a fascial ligament, while the posterior layer should be referred to as a neurovascular bundle consisting of the subureteral tissue. To excise the anterior layer, scissors are inserted along the medial aspect of the ureter to the entrance of the ureteric tunnel (panel (**a**) of Fig. 2.25), creating a tunnel. Manipulation to incise the created roof of the ureteric tunnel is repeated two or three times. The space created by excision of the anterior layer is called the paravaginal space. After freeing the ureter, the posterior layer is separated and excised by inserting scissors from the paravaginal space toward the paravesical space (panel (**b**)). Unfortunately, Okabayashi did not provide any description of the microscopic anatomy of the posterior layer.

Okabayashi's anterior manipulation systematically implemented excision of CL from the Clark/Wertheim procedure (Fig. 2.12) by adding depth to the excision. Furthermore, to separate the entire Mackenrodt ligament, the paravaginal space was excavated down to the pelvic floor, so that it can be presumed that the entire posterior layer was separated and excised between the paravaginal and paravesical spaces (Fig. 3.18). However, Fig. 2.7 does not show that the excavation extends to the lower portion of the pararectal space.

3.1.2 The Latzko Procedure (Peham and Amreich 1930)

In Latzko's anterior manipulation, the handling of the medial and lateral aspects of the ureter is entirely different in exposing all the layers of the Mackenrodt ligament. Manipulation of the medial aspect of the ureter involves excision of the bladder pillar by the Wertheim procedure with the ureter slightly shifted laterally (Figs. 2.12 and 2.26).

In contrast, as shown in panel (**a**) of Fig. 2.4, manipulation of the lateral aspect of the ureter involves excavation of the paravesical space down to the pelvic floor, exposing the levator ani muscle. To carry out complete excision of the Mackenrodt ligament, or TCL including the lateral rectal ligament, in the Latzko procedure, the entire anterior aspect of the ligament must first be exposed. However, manipulation of the medial aspect of the ureter by the Wertheim procedure did not reach the pelvic floor. Even Latzko did not describe how to reach the pelvic floor for this manipulation. So, the author infers the following solution for it.

The lateral pelvic ligament, or SS, represented in panel (**a**) of Fig. 2.27, is composed of the following: (a) the paravesical space (colored pink) on the lateral aspect of the ureter to be excavated down to the pelvic floor; (b) Okabayashi's paravaginal space or author's fourth space to be excavated on the medial aspect of the ureter (colored blue); and (c) underlying tissue between two spaces (colored yellow), which is contiguous with the ureter corresponding to the posterior layer of Okabayashi's vesicouterine ligament or author's anterior mesoureter.

Panel (**b**) represents tissue image of SS created centering around the ureter with its underlying tissue. Further details of this tissue image will be discussed in the section on the anterior parametrium (pp. 75–76).

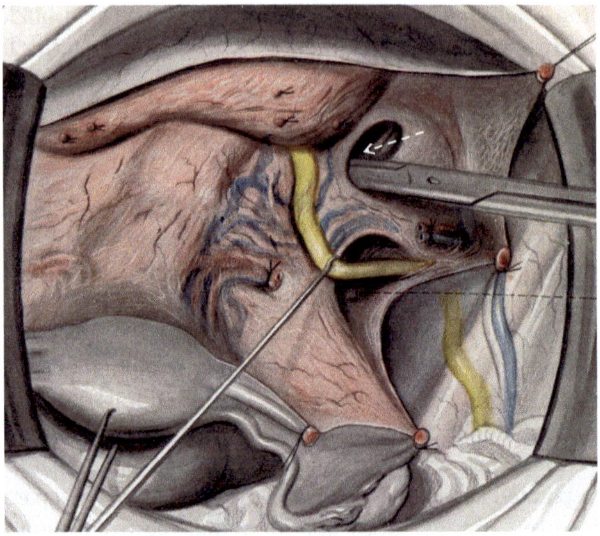

Peham-Amreich, 1930

Fig. 2.26 Handling of the vesicouterine ligament in the Latzko procedure
Figure 2.12 of P&A shows the vesicouterine ligament has been excised but does not represent a complete excision of the Okabayashi's vesicouterine ligament. There is no explicit mention of the Wertheim procedure in P&A's surgical manual. The author speculates that the reason for this is as follows: In P&A's surgical manual stated on p. 347, Fig. 206: "The connective tissue capsule of the paravesical fat is pierced with the scissors just behind the bulge of the bladder and the fat is pushed to the side." It is believed that, in P&A's procedure, scissors are inserted from the developed paravesical space shown in Fig. 2.26 in a direction of the dashed white arrow, breaking through tissue, or anterior mesoureter, that corresponds to the posterior layer of Okabayashi, then entering tissue on the medial aspect of the ureter

The route of entry into the medial aspect of the ureter, or blue portion in panel (**a**) of Fig. 2.27, can be inferred from the following passage in P&A's surgical manual (Peham 1934, Fig. 206, p. 347): "The connective tissue capsule of the paravesical fat is pierced with the scissors just behind the bulge of the bladder, and the fat is pushed to the side." In other words, the author considers that, as seen in Fig. 2.26, scissors were inserted from the paravesical space penetrating through Okabayashi's posterior layer as depicted by arrows in panels (**a**) and (**b**) of Fig. 2.27. Ultimately, excluding the ureter, the blue portion and neural and vascular regions, or posterior layer, running along the boundary would be excised.

In conclusion, regardless of the merits of each surgical procedure, the anterior manipulation of the Latzko and Okabayashi procedures ultimately results in the same state. In short, both procedures achieve the complete exposure of the entire anterior aspect of the Mackenrodt ligament through excavation of the entire paravesical space, but at the cost of inadvertently excising blood vessels and nerves to/from the bladder (Figs. 3.10 and 3.24).

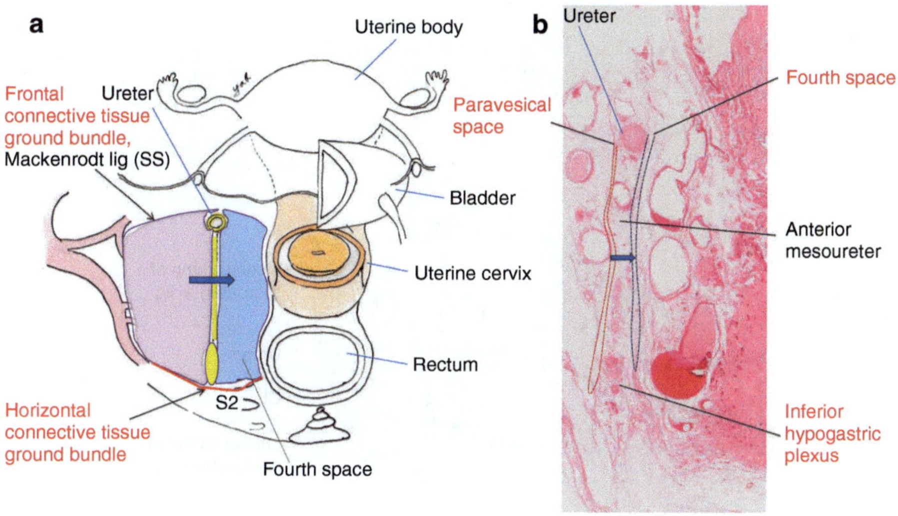

Fig. 2.27 Method of exposure for entire anterior surface of the Mackenrodt ligament in the Latzko procedure

A schematic illustration and a histological sample show details of the procedure. Viewed anteriorly, panel (**a**) depicts the pelvic organs and classical lateral parametrium, or *TCL including the lateral rectal ligament* (so called Mackenrodt ligament). The lateral parametrium (pink) represents the paravesical space that has been excavated down to the pelvic floor, while the blue area, which is designated as the author's fourth space, represents the unexcavated portion. The frontal connective tissue ground bundle refers to the classical lateral parametrium, or TCL including the lateral rectal ligament, while the horizontal connective tissue ground bundle (red line) indicates Mackenrodt's short fibrous bundle, or the superior fascia of the levator ani muscle

Panel (**b**) depicts a histological tissue image by frontal dissection from a cadaver with focus on the area in yellow corresponding to the boundary between the pink and blue regions in panel (**a**). The neurovascular bundle sandwiched between the paravesical and fourth spaces corresponds to the anterior mesoureter. Further details on this tissue sample are shown in Fig. 3.16. P&A's procedure involves perforating the anterior mesoureter with scissors from the excavated paravesical space (pink area in panel (**a**)) in a direction shown by the arrow so as to enter the fourth space (blue area in panel (**a**)). This is followed by excision of the anterior mesoureter and tissue that fills the fourth space, thereby fully exposing the anterior surface of the Mackenrodt ligament

3.2 *Posterior Manipulation*

3.2.1 The Okabayashi Procedure

In the Okabayashi procedure, the posterior manipulation is carried out at the beginning of surgery. After incising the Douglas pouch and creating the rectovaginal pouch, the uterosacral ligament is severed (red area in Fig. 2.28). From the gap between the two severed ends, the procedure progresses caudally along the sacral surface and laterally along the posterior surface of the parametrium, while excising the areolar connective tissue and then developing the pararectal space (yellow arrow in Fig. 2.28).

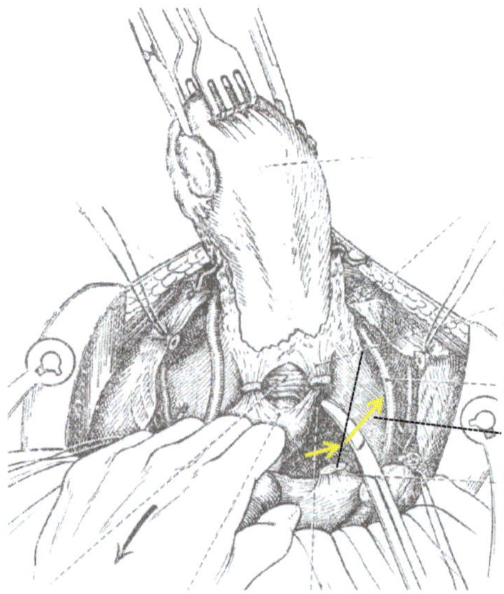

Fig. 2.28 Development of the pararectal space according to Okabayashi's procedure
Okabayashi described reaching the anterior surface of the sacrum as follows: Approaching from the space between the medial and lateral stumps of the uterosacral ligament, create and expand it further anteriorly and laterally while cutting through the loose connective tissue on the posterior aspect of the lateral parametrium (yellow arrows). (Reproduced from Okabayashi 1952b, Fig. 17, p. 22, in Japanese)

3.2.2 The Latzko Procedure

In contrast to the Okabayashi procedure, the posterior manipulation in Latzko's is carried out toward the end of surgery. The posterior portion of the ureter is separated, followed by development of the upper portion of the pararectal space from a lateral to medial aspect, that is, from the pelvic sidewall toward the uterosacral ligament, opposite to Okabayashi's manipulation.

In conclusion, in both the Latzko and Okabayashi procedures, the posterior manipulation involves freeing the ureter. However, to expose the entire posterior surface of the Mackenrodt ligament, the hypogastric nerves and blood vessels must also be excised, theoretically resulting in the same state as for the anterior manipulation.

3.3 Lateral Manipulation (Conventional Parametrectomy)

In both the Latzko and Okabayashi procedures, despite differences in their surgical approaches, the Mackenrodt ligament, or TCL including the lateral rectal ligament, is ultimately exposed on its entire anterior and posterior surfaces before being excised theoretically. It can be said that L&S and Okabayashi were not aware of the lateral rectal ligament. Naturally, there is no description given regarding the contradiction in the procedure where TCL and the lateral rectal ligament shown in Fig. 2.20 are excised en bloc. As shown in panel (**a**) of Fig. 2.8, P&A excise the rectal pillar or superior fascia of levator ani along with the Mackenrodt ligament. However, no such description is found in Okabayashi's surgical manual.

3.3.1 Peham & Amreich's Parametrectomy (Panel (a) of Fig. 2.8)

P&A described the separation and excision of the Mackenrodt ligament as follows (Peham 1934, pp. 346–8): "In inserting the finger from the upper chamber of the pararectal space into the combined spaces it should pass along the sacrospinous ligament and the coccygeus muscle in a direction forward, downward and laterally. The finger thus raises the base of the Mackenrodt ligament from the levator. By this method of dissection, the Mackenrodt ligament is laid free anteriorly, posteriorly, below and above. Two clamps are placed on the ligament, one near the pelvic wall and second mesial to it and the structure is divided between the clamps. The lateral clamp must be applied so that its tip extends beyond the base of the Mackenrodt ligament and lies in the canal artificially made with the finger." The results of this parametrectomy are depicted in panel (**a**) of Fig. 2.8 and panel (**b**) of Fig. 2.9. The author himself has had no experience in extended endopelvic resection. In the time when an extensive and radical approach overlapped, it is likely that there were some skilled practitioners who must have mastered such techniques. Furthermore, it is evident that the lateral rectal ligament was not recognized as shown in panel (**b**) of Fig. 2.9. However, this knowledge gained regarding the existence of the rectal pillar was useful for the combined excision of the rectum.

3.3.2 Okabayashi's Parametrectomy

In this procedure, while excavating the paravaginal/paravesical and pararectal spaces, the fascia of the Mackenrodt ligament is simultaneously excised. As a result, the thinned Mackenrodt ligament is separated and severed by perforation of both the paravesical and pararectal spaces (red arrow in panel (**a**) of Fig. 2.29). While the specific site, where both spaces are connected, is not explicitly stated, but in panel (**b**), the tip of the clamped lateral forceps can be seen located near the pelvic floor. The Okabayashi procedure is not an extended endopelvic fascial resection like that in the Latzko procedure.

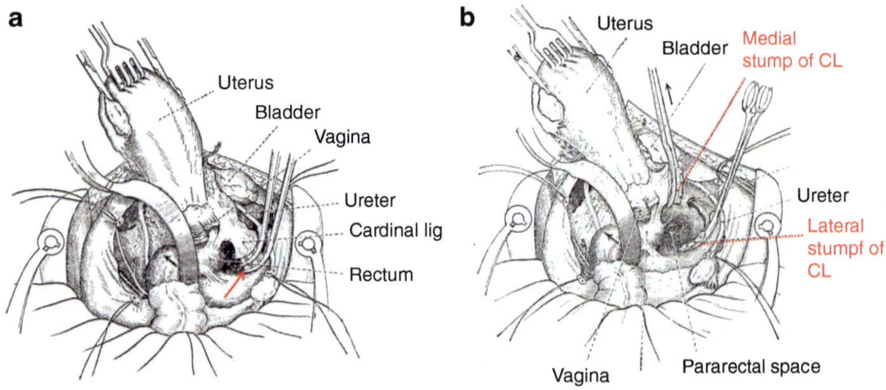

Fig. 2.29 Okabayashi's handling of TCL
Panel (**a**) depicts the excised fascia of this ligament, with the TCL reduced in size and clamped near the pelvic wall
Panel (**b**) shows the condition after excision of the ligament. The tips of the clamps are seen to reach the pelvic floor. The excision of TCL in Fig. 2.8 seems to have followed Okabayashi's procedure. (Reproduced from Okabayashi 1952b; Figs. 2.19 and 2.27, pp. 22 and 28, in Japanese)

4 Paracolpium and Paracolpectomy

No detailed anatomy of the paracolpium and corresponding method for its excision are to be found for RH. As depicted in Fig. 2.4, it appears that parametrectomy has been carried out with a "do as you please."

The paracolpium in the Latzko procedure resembles DeLancey's level I (suspension) (DeLancy 1992). Okabayashi's concept of the paracolpium refers only to the neurovascular bundle on the medial aspect of the tendinous arch of the pelvic fascia, which is similar to DeLancey's level II (attachment). The superior fascia of the levator ani muscle is excised in the Latzko's procedure but is not targeted for excision in the Okabayashi procedure. Following is a discussion on paracolpectomy.

4.1 Paracolpectomy in the Latzko Procedure

In panel (**b**) of Fig. 2.9, the rectal pillar has been excised, exposing the levator ani muscle. This finding suggests that Latzko's procedure for paracolpectomy may have involved the excision of the parietal endopelvic fascia. This endopelvic fascia corresponds to the superior fascia of the levator ani muscle, which Mackenrodt in 1895 referred to as a short fibrous bundle and described it as follows: "Short fibrous bundles arise from the fascia of the levator ani as a sort of inferior continuation of the transverse cervical ligament and attach to the side of the connective tissue sheath surrounding the vagina, thus providing further support" (Mackenrodt 1895; Speert

1996). Also, from panel (**a**) of Fig. 2.4 in which the levator ani muscle is seen exposed, it can be concluded that the short fibrous bundle was included as a target for paracolpectomy in the Latzko procedure. In panel (**b**), the relationship between the short fibrous bundle and horizontal connective tissue ground bundle is not clearly defined.

4.2 Paracolpectomy in the Okabayashi Procedure

Okabayashi described that the lateral vaginal tissue, or paracolpium, is continuous with the stump of the TCL and appears (Fig. 2.30) in the space, namely, the combined space of the paravaginal and paravesical spaces, created by the severance of the posterior layer of the vesicouterine ligament.

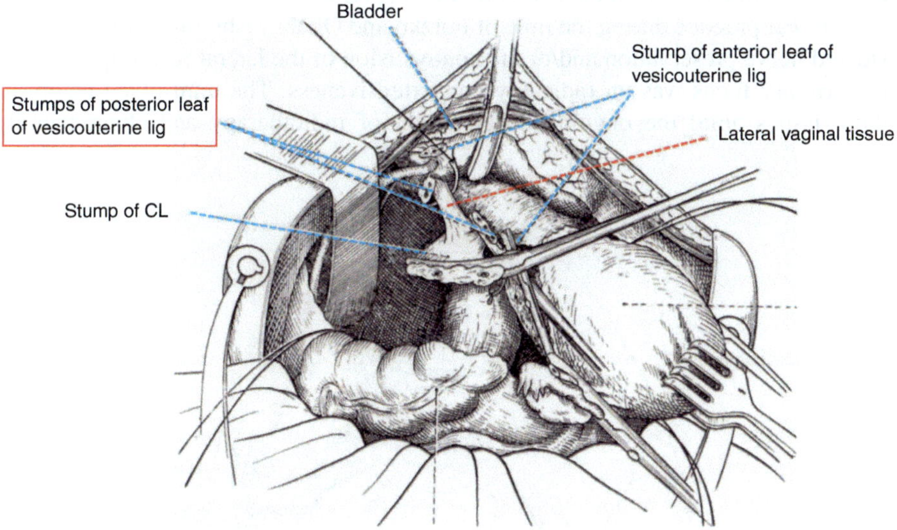

Fig. 2.30 Exposure of lateral vaginal tissue according to Okabayashi
Okabayashi describes that, upon excision of the posterior layer of the vesicouterine ligament, the deep caudal portion reveals the lateral vaginal tissue, which continues from the visceral edge of TCL. The author agrees with this view of Okabayashi's paracolpium. The fascia of the levator ani muscle is not excised together with the paracolpium. This figure depicts a needle passing through the paravaginal tissue at a level where severance of the vaginal canal is to be carried out. (Reproduced from Okabayashi 1952b, Fig. 28, p. 35, in Japanese)

By enlarging this combined space caudally, the lateral vaginal tissue becomes fully exposed and excised. Okabayashi's combined space is considered to correspond to the space formed at the junction between Mackenrodt's short fibrous bundle and the connective tissue sheath surrounding the vagina.

5 Summary of the Latzko and Okabayashi Procedures

P&A's Latzko procedure in 1930 is more complex in terms of procedure compared to Okabayashi's in 1952 and difficult to apply in current practice. This could be due to the difference of more than 20 years between their publications. It is conceivable that Okabayashi and P&A mutually influenced each other. For example, P&A stated in the anatomy section of their surgical manual, "This term (vesico-uterine ligament) is not essentially correct, because this structure does not, as the name implies, extend to the uterus, but to the Mackenrodt ligament." This statement suggests that P&A may have drawn inspiration from Okabayashi's article in 1921 (Okabayashi 1921). However, it was never put into practical use. The author also believes that Okabayashi's idea regarding the blood vessels of the posterior layer in 1952 may have been influenced to some extent by P&A (Fig. 2.31).

Surgical practice during the time of Latzko and Okabayashi might not have considered nerve preservation and/or the non-excision of the lateral rectal ligament, as the primary focus was on radicality and extensiveness. The unresolved nature of these issues amid the ongoing development of radiotherapy and chemotherapy

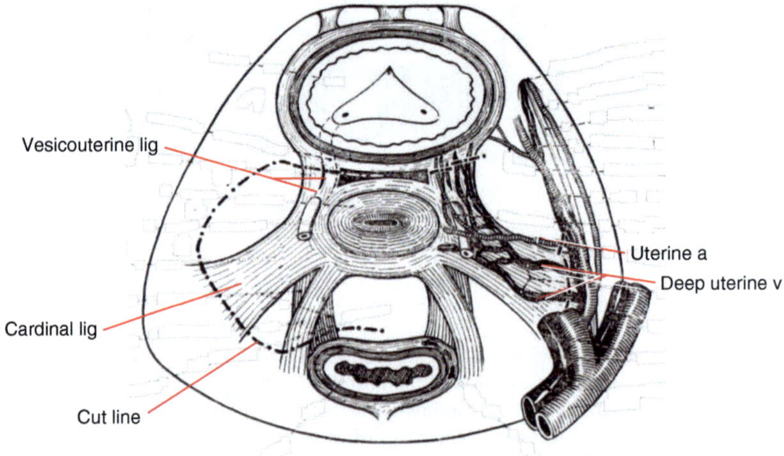

Fig. 2.31 Pathway of vessels within the parametrium according to Okabayashi
Okabayashi clearly recognized the vascular connection between the vesicouterine ligament and TCL. Here, the veins that drain from the bladder to the deep uterine vein are depicted. (Reproduced from Okabayashi 1952b, Fig. 3, p. 8, in Japanese)

continued until the late twentieth century and may have contributed to the decline in today's surgical treatment of cervical cancer in the West. However, the author believes that L&S, Okabayashi, P&A, and Meigs must have influenced each other to some degree in the shaping of an original form of procedure for RH in the twentieth century. We must earnestly confront their achievements in RH and search for a surgical procedure that meets a standard of QOL fitting for the twenty-first century.

References

Averette HE, Nguyen HN, Donato DM et al (1993) Radical hysterectomy for invasive cervical cancer: a 25-year prospective experience with the Miami technique. Cancer Suppl 71:1422–1437. PMID: 8431876. https://doi.org/10.1002/cncr.2820710407

Cibula D, Abu-Rustum NR, Benedetti-Panici P et al (2011) New classification system of radical hysterectomy: emphasis on a three-dimensional anatomic template for parametrial resection. Gynecol Oncol 122:264–268. PMID: 21592548. Epub 2011 May 17. https://doi.org/10.1016/j.ygyno.2011.04.029

Clark JG (1895) A more radical method of performing hysterectomy for cancer of the uterus. Johns Hopkins Hosp Bull 6:120–124

Curtis AH, Anson BJ, Beaton LE (1940) The anatomy of the subperitoneal tissues and ligamentous structures in relation to surgery of the female pelvic viscera. Surg Gyn Obst 70:643–656

DeLancy JOL (1992) Anatomic aspects of vaginal eversion after hysterectomy. Am J Obstet Gynecol 166:1717–1728. PMID: 1615980. https://doi.org/10.1016/0002-9378(92)91562-o

Enker WE, Thaler HT, Cranor ML et al (1995) Total mesorectal excision in the operative treatment of carcinoma of the rectum. J Am Coll Surg 181:335–346. PMID: 7551328

Heald RJ (1988) The 'holy plane' of rectal surgery. J R Soc Med 81:503–508. PMID: 3184105, PMCID: PMC1291757. https://doi.org/10.1177/014107688808100904

Heald RJ, Husband EM, Ryall RD (1982) The mesorectum in rectal surgery. Brit J Surg 69:613–616. PMID: 6751457. https://doi.org/10.1002/bjs.1800691019

Höckel M (1999) Laterally extended endopelvic resection: surgical treatment of infrailiac pelvic wall recurrences of gynecologic malignancies. Am J Obstet Gynecol 180:306–312. PMID: 9988791. https://doi.org/10.1016/s0002-9378(99)70204-8

Höckel M (2007) Total mesometrial resection: new concept for radical hysterectomy based on developmentally defined compartments of local tumor spread. In: The 16th annual review course on gynecologic oncology and pathology, Kyoto, Japan

Höckel M, Horn LC, Hentschel B et al (2003) Total mesometrial resection: high resolution nerve-sparing radical hysterectomy based on developmentally defined surgical anatomy. Int J Gynecol Cancer 13:791–803. PMID: 14675316. https://doi.org/10.1111/j.1525-1438.2003.13608.x

Höckel M, Horn LC, Fritsch H (2005) Association between the mesenchymal compartment of uterovaginal organogenesis and local tumor spread in stage IB-IIB cervical carcinoma: a prospective study. Lancet Oncol 6:751–756. PMID: 16198980. https://doi.org/10.1016/S1470-2045(05)70324-7

Höckel M, Horn LC, Manthey N et al (2009) Resection of the embryologically defined uterovaginal (Müllerian) compartment and pelvic control in patients with cervical cancer: a prospective analysis. Lancet Oncol 10(7):683–692. PMID: 19482513. https://doi.org/10.1016/S1470-2045(09)70100-7

Hoshiba T, Yabuki Y, Asamoto A et al (2000) Our laporoscopic radical hysterectomy. Gynecol Obstet Surg 11:93–100. (in Japanese)

Kobayashi T (1961) Abdominal radical hysterectomy with pelvic lymphadenectomy for cancer of the cervix. Nanzando, Tokyo. (in Japanese)

Kocks J (1880) Die Normale und Pathologische Lage und Gestalt des Uterus Sowie deren Mechanik. Max Cohen & Sohn, Bonn

Latzko W, Schiffmann J (1919) Zur Radikaloperation des Gebarmutterkrebses. 361 Diskussinsbemerkungen. Zbl Gynäk 43:689–698

Mackenrodt A (1895) Ueber die Ursachen der normalen und pathologischen Lagen des Uterus. Arch F Gynäk 48:393–421

Magrina JF, Pawlina W, Kho RM et al (2011) Robotic nerve-sparing radical hysterectomy: feasibility and technique. Gynecol Oncol 121:605–609. PMID: 21419478. https://doi.org/10.1016/j.ygyno.2011.02.034

Meigs JV (1945) Wertheim operation for carcinoma of cervix. Am J Obstet Gynecol 49:542–553

Meigs JV (1954) Radical hysterectomy with bilateral dissection of the pelvic lymph nodes. In: Meigs JV (ed) Surgical treatment of cancer of the cervix. Grune Stratton, New York, pp 149–216

Miles EE (1908) A method of performing abdomino-perineal excision for carcinoma of the rectum and of the terminal portion of the pelvic colon. Lancet 2:1812–1813

Monk BJ, Toita T, Wu X et al (2023) Durvalumab versus placebo with chemoradiotherapy for locally advanced cervical cancer (CALLA): a randomized, double-blind, phase 3 trial. Lancet Oncol 24(12):1334–1348. https://doi.org/10.1016/S1470-2045(23)00479-5. PMID: 38039991

Moriya Y, Hojo K, Sawada T, Koyama Y (1989) Significance of lateral node dissection for advanced rectal carcinoma at or below the peritoneal reflection. Dis Col Rect 32:307–315

Netter FH (2006) Atlas of human anatomy, 4th edn. Saunders

Okabayashi H (1921) Radical abdominal hysterectomy for cancer of cervix uteri. Surg Gynecol Obstet 33:335–341

Okabayashi H (1952a) Systematic abdominal radical hysterectomy for cancer of cervix uteri. Tokyo, Kanehara. (in Japanese)

Okabayashi H (1952b) Radical operation for cancer of uterine cervix. Tokyo, Kanehara

Oosterhuis JW, Lung PF, Verschueren RCJ et al (1985) Viability of tumor cells in the irrigation fluid of the cavitron ultrasonic surgical aspirator (CUSA) after tumor fragmentation. Cancer 56:368–370. PMID:4005801. https://doi.org/10.1002/1097-0142(19850715)56:2<368:aid-cncr2820560227>3.0.co;2-4

Peham HV, Amreich J (1930) Gynäkologische Operationslehre. Verlag S. Karger, Berlin/Basel

Peham HV, Amreich J (1934) Operative gynecology, vol. 2 (translated by Ferguson LK). JB Lippincott, Philadelphia, pp 333–366

Pernkopf E (1943) Topographische Anatomie des Menschen. Zweiter Band. Urban und Schwarzenberg, Berlin

Piver MS, Rutledge F, Smith JP (1974) Five classes of extended hysterectomy for women with cervical cancer. Obstet Gynecol 44:265–271. PMID: 4417035. [PubMed] [Google Scholar]

Plante M, Kwon JS, Ferguson S, Samouëlian V, Ferron G et al (2024) Simple versus radical hysterectomy in women with low-risk cervical cancer. N Engl J Med 390:819–829. https://doi.org/10.1056/NEJMoa2308900

Platzer W (ed) (1989) Pernkopf anatomy: atlas of topographic and applied human anatomy, vol II: thorax, abdomen and extremities, 3rd edn. Urban Schwarzenberg, Baltimore/Munich

Querleu D, Morrow CP (2008) Classification of radical hysterectomy. Lancet Oncol 9:297–303. PMID:18308255. https://doi.org/10.1016/S1470-2045(08)70074-3

Ramirez PT, Frumovitz M, Pareja R et al (2018) Minimally invasive versus abdominal radical hysterectomy for cervical cancer. N Engl J Med 379:1895–1904. PMID: 30380365. https://doi.org/10.1056/NEJMoa1806395

Reiffenstuhl G (1982) The clinical significance of the connective tissue planes and spaces. Clin Obstet Gynecol 25:812–820

Rose PG, Bundy BN, Watkins EB et al (1999) Concurrent cisplatin-based radiotherapy and chemotherapy for locally advanced cervical cancer. N Engl J Med 340:1144–1153. PMID: 10202165. https://doi.org/10.1056/NEJM199904153401502

Savage H (1870) The surgery, surgical pathology, and surgical anatomy of the female pelvic organ, 3rd edn. J & A Churchill & Son, London, p 76

Savage H (1880) The surgery, surgical pathology and surgical anatomy of the female pelvic organs. William Wood & Co, New York

Speert H (1996) Obstetrics and gynecologic milestones illustrated. Parthenon, New York, pp 138–141

Sugihara K, Kobayashi H, Kato T et al (2006) Indication and benefit of pelvic sidewall dissection for rectal cancer. Dis Colon Rectum 49:1663–1672. PMID: 17041749

Uhlenhuth E, Day DE, Smith RD et al (1948) The visceral endopelvic fascia and the hypogastric sheath. Surg Gynecol Obstet 86:9–28. PMID: 18920874

Verleye I, Vergot I, Reed N et al (2009) Quality assurance for radical hysterectomy for cervical cancer: the view of the European Organization for Research and Treatment of Cancer-Gynecological Cancer Group (EORTC-GCG). Ann Oncol 20:1631–1638

Wertheim E (1911) Die erweiterte abdominale Operation bei Carcinoma colli uteri (auf Grund von 500 Fällen). Urban & Schwarzenberg, Berlin, pp 356–357

Wertheim E (1912) The extended abdominal operation for carcinoma uteri (based on 500 operative cases). Am J Obstet Dis Women Child 66:169–232

Yabuki Y (1997) Cardinal ligament dissection based on a new theory. CEM. J Gynecol Oncol 2:278–287. [Google Scholar]

Yabuki Y (2019) New radical hysterectomy for uterine cancer. In: Theory and technique for nerve-sparing operation, 3rd edn. Medical View, Tokyo. (in Japanese with figure legend in English)

Yabuki Y (2023) Two lateral parametria in radical hysterectomy: history and outcome. J Obstet Gynecol Res. 43:1069–1078

Yabuki Y, Asamoto A, Hoshiba T et al (1991) Dissection of the cardinal ligament in radical hysterectomy for cervical cancer with emphasis on the lateral ligament. Am J Obstet Gynec 164:7–14. PMID: 1986630. https://doi.org/10.1016/0002-9378(91)90614-w

Yabuki Y, Asamoto A, Hoshiba T et al (2000) Radical hysterectomy: an anatomic evaluation of parametrial dissection. Gynecol Oncol 77:155–163. PMID: 10739705. https://doi.org/10.1006/gyno.1999

Yabuki Y, Sasaki H, Hatakeyama N et al (2005) Discrepancies between classic anatomy and modern gynecologic surgery on pelvic connective tissue structure: harmonization of those concepts by collaborative cadaver dissection. Am J Obstet Gynecol 193:7–15. PMID: 16021052. https://doi.org/10.1016/j.ajog.2005.02.108

Yabuki Y et al (2011) Redefinition of the pelvic connective tissue: in-situ histologic examination. Female Pelvic Med & Reconstr Surg 17:60–66

Chapter 3
Author's Clinical Anatomy

Abbreviations

CL	Cardinal ligament
IFFA	International Federation of Associations of Anatomists
IHP	Inferior hypogastric plexus
L&S	Latzko and Schiffmann
LP	Lateral parametrium
LUL	Lateral umbilical ligament
NSRH	Nerve-sparing radical hysterectomy
P&A	Peham-Americh
PSN	Pelvic splanchnic nerve
Q&M	Querleu and Morrow
RH	Radical hysterectomy
TA	Terminologia Anatomica
TCL	Transverse cervical ligament
TMMR	Total mesometrial resection
VUL	Vesicouterine ligament

The goal for twenty-first century RH must meet specific requirements that impart minimum stress on the body and, at the same time, preserve bodily functions. To achieve this, the twentieth century surgical concept of RH must be reestablished and based on one capable of accommodating the morphological changes on a body induced by surgical manipulations. By coining a term "*clinical anatomy*" that would form the foundation of this new surgical concept, the author will discuss in this chapter his perspective on reconciling patient's safety with surgical procedures.

Y. Yabuki, *Nerve-Sparing Radical Hysterectomy*,
https://doi.org/10.1007/978-981-96-7194-6_3

1 Discourse on Artificial Spaces

The principle of surgery for uterine cervical cancer involves, whenever possible, complete excision of the carcinomatous lesion. This, however, must be compatible with preservation of the function of the surrounding organs. To accomplish this, ligaments that are separated for creating artificial spaces in a living body must be selectively excised.

Figure 3.1 shows a simulated dissection for RH on a fresh cadaver. Here, four spaces can be seen excavated: the paravesical space, fourth space, Latzko's pararectal space, and Okabayashi's pararectal space. This excavation allows for the dissection of the bundle, or *supporting system (SS),* consisting of the visceral vessels passing from the internal iliac vessels (Fig. 2.20). Also dissected is the lamina, or *mesoureter*, composed of vessels and pelvic autonomic nerves hanging from the ureter (panel (**b**) of Fig. 2.27). During this surgical procedure, the vessels to be excised are selectively separated from SS and the mesoureter.

Based on Fig. 3.1, four spaces can be seen excavated in the loose connective tissue of a fixed cadaver in Fig. 3.2 and are developed perpendicularly to the organs, and the two emerged bundles surgically verified to intersect at approximately a right angle.

Figure 3.3 depicts the relationship between spaces and ligaments created in the lesser pelvic cavity based on cadaver dissections shown in Figs. 3.1 and 3.2 and

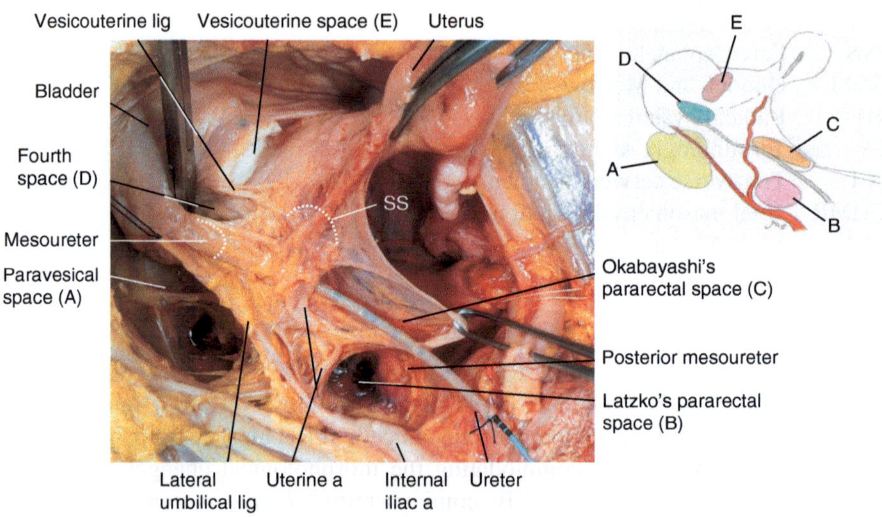

Fig. 3.1 Artificial spaces created during radical hysterectomy
Direction of the spaces excavated during RH is classified into two: one being perpendicular to the uterus, which includes paravesical, fourth, Latzko's pararectal, and Okabayashi's pararectal spaces, and the other horizontal to the uterus and vagina, which includes vesicouterine/vaginal pouch and rectouterine/vaginal pouch. The excavation of these spaces leads to the separation of TCL, the mesoureter, and vesicouterine and uterosacral ligaments. (Reproduced from Yabuki 2020)

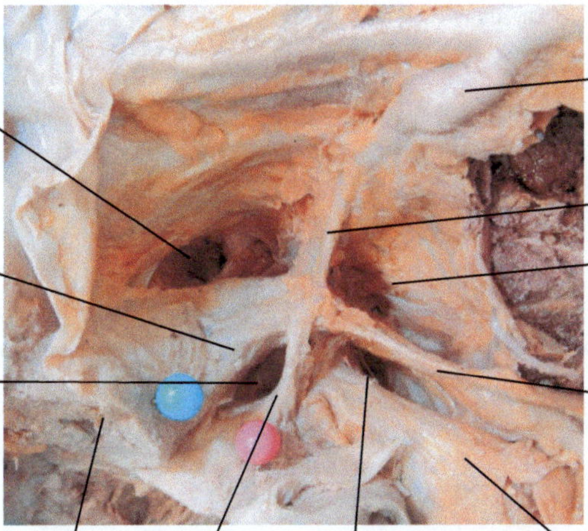

Fig. 3.2 Artificial spaces excavated in the right subserous layer
This photograph almost from a bird's-eye-view focuses on the right side of the pelvis oriented toward a cranial aspect of a fixed cadaver. It shows the four perpendicularly excavated spaces: the paravesical space, fourth space, Latzko's pararectal space, and Okabayashi's pararectal space, and the structures separated by these spaces including SS and mesoureter

demonstrated in surgery in Figs. 2.13, 2.18, 2.19, and 2.20. Illustrations in Fig. 2.1 and Fig. 2.3 by P&A and author, respectively, imply that these surgically excavated spaces are perpendicular to the organs, not horizontal.

Although the paravesical space can easily be excavated adjacent to the urogenital hiatus, it is not required for RH. The pararectal space terminates adjacent to S3 without advancing caudally. The two bundles that are intersected and divided by SS and the mesoureter, both depicted in Fig. 3.1, are respectively designated as the lateral and medial supporting systems and anterior and posterior mesoureters.

Figure 3.4 is a diagrammatic cross section of the pelvis frequently cited by P&A (Fig. 132 in Peham and Amreich 1934, p. 180) taken from panels (**a**) of Figs. 2.1 and 2.3 by P&A and author, respectively. However, it does not correspond with the cross section of the Mackenrodt ligament, or *TCL including the lateral rectal ligament*, shown in Kobayashi's Fig. 2.6, Pernkopf's Fig. 2.14, and/or the author's Figs. 2.20 and 2.34, demonstrating the relationship between the uterus and rectum orientated perpendicular. If Fig. 3.4 depicts a frontal cross section as demonstrated, the lateral rectal ligament must be drawn in the pararectal space (Fig. 2.17). Even today, this figure continues to be cited in many surgical manuals. Nevertheless, disparity between P&A's surgical procedure and their anatomy observed in panel (**a**) of Fig. 2.1 and panels (**b**) and (**a**) of Fig. 2.4 is also apparent in Fig. 3.4. At this point, one can imagine their distress regarding the gap between basic anatomy and clinical evidence of the 1930s. Details concerning this will be discussed in the following section.

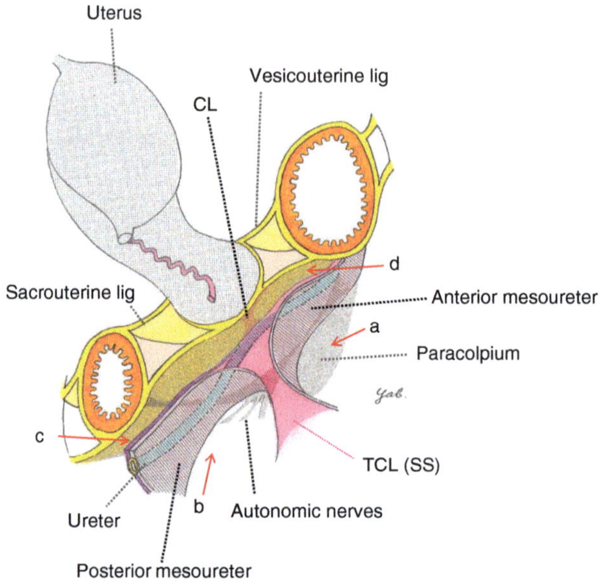

Fig. 3.3 Schematic illustration of pelvic connective tissue and spaces
In an attempt to classify the subserous layer based on pelvic connective tissue and spaces, Figs. 3.1 and 3.2 were combined to form a model schematic illustration in Fig. 3.3. The ligaments that connect the pelvic organs to the pelvic sidewall are referred to as SS, and the lamina extending along the ureters is called the mesoureter, as has already been mentioned. The region where the two bundles intersect can tentatively be referred to as the anterior and posterior mesoureters and lateral and medial supporting systems, respectively. When applied to TCL, this region should be referred to as the lateral and medial TCL. If the uterine broad ligament is drawn covering the ascending uterine vessels, it would complete the illustration. (Reproduced from Yabuki et al. 2005)

2 Clinical Anatomy of the Lateral Support or Supporting System

2.1 Overview

In the sixth edition of Nomina Anatomica in 1980, the only anatomic terms that related to the lateral parametrium of the uterus were the Lig. Latum uteri and Parametrium. In 1998, Terminologia Anatomica (ed. Tieme) introduced new anatomic terms of paracervix, pubocervical ligament, cardinal ligament, transverse cervical ligament, uterosacral ligament, and recto-uterine ligament. Of these, CL and TCL were adopted as synonymous, as were the uterosacral and rectouterine ligaments. This revision is somewhat inconsistent. For example, without the use of terms such as the paravesical and pararectal spaces, TCL cannot be explained. In addition, Savage/Kocks' CL and Mackenrodt's TCL are not synonymous and must therefore be distinguished both historically and surgically (Mackenrodt 1895;

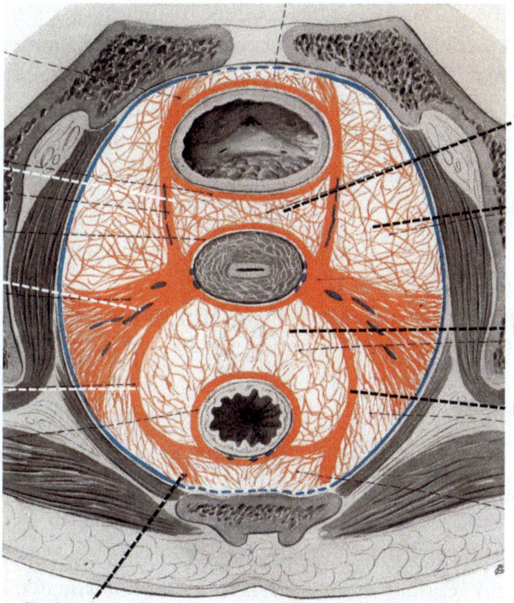

Fig. 3.4 Diagrammatic cross section of the pelvis by P&A. (Reproduced from Peham and Amreich 1930, Fig. 132 , p. 191)
This diagram strongly suggests that the lateral ligament of the genitalia is parallel to the lateral border of the genitalia, and that the paravesical and pararectal spaces have a horizontal relationship with the lateral ligament of the genitalia. However, the genitalia in this context refers to the vagina, and the lateral ligament of the genitalia refers to the paracolpium. This cannot be applied to the uterine cervix and parametrium (Fig. 2.27)

Savage 1870; Kocks 1880). Moreover, it is not clear what the introduced paracervix in the 12th edition represents.

Throughout the history of surgery for cervical cancer, the lack of established conventions for naming surgically altered anatomic forms has led to multiple terms for the same form, resulting in a great deal of confusion. One such example is the CL (of Mackenrodt).

From the mid-twentieth century, the concept of "CL (of Mackenrodt)," was used by Uhlenhuth et al. (1948) and Reiffenstuhl (1982). It was also adopted in the 30th American edition of Gray's Anatomy in 1985 (Clemente 1985) with a part of the description as follows: "CL (of Mackenrodt) is a fibrous sheet of the subserous fascia embedded in the adipose tissue on each side of the lower cervix uteri and vagina. To form it, the fasciae over the ventral and dorsal walls of the vagina and cervix come together at the lateral border of these organs and the resulting sheet extends across the pelvic floor as a deeper continuation of the broad ligament." This description is precisely represented in Fig. 2.1. As far as the author knows, this basic concept first appeared in the 15th edition of Gray's Anatomy (Pick and Howden 1901) as follows: "The two lateral or broad ligaments pass from the sides of the uterus to the lateral walls of the pelvis, …" This concept further evolved into the concept of CL by Savage/Kocks. This heritage has been consistently handed down by noted surgeons such as P&A (Fig. 2.1), Howkins in Bonny's Gynecological Surgery in 1974 (Howkins and Stallworthy 1974), Netter (panel (**a**) of Fig. 2.3), as well as in today's Mayo Clinic's Magrina (Magrina et al. 2011), and by Q&M, and Cibula's group (Cibula et al. 2011). These terms have also continued to be handed down in the following literature:

1. Gray's Anatomy: Deeper continuation of the broad ligament (30th American ed.; p. 1575) (Clemente 1985)
2. Greenhill Obstetrics: Enhancement of lowermost aspects of the broad ligament (p. 110, 1974) (Greenhill and Friedman. 1974)
3. TeLinde Gynecologic Surgery: The base of the broad ligament (8th ed.; p. 1468) (Rock and Thompson 1996)

Meanwhile, the 36th British edition of Gray's Anatomy in 1980 mentioned the TCL (of Mackenrodt) as well as, separately, the existence of the lateral ligament of the rectum.

Today's gynecologists carrying out RH have seen the emergence of various surgical instruments and technological advancements, but since the presentation of L&S and Okabayashi procedures that were based on Mackenrodt's TCL theory, no new surgical techniques based on new theories have emerged (Höckel's TMMR is not considered as an RH.). One of the reasons for this is synonymization of CL and TCL (Yabuki et al. 1991). As mentioned earlier, CL is a longitudinal and horizontal structure on the medial aspect of the ureter, whereas TCL is a transversal and perpendicular structure on both the medial and lateral aspects of the ureter, forming a continuum with the lateral rectal ligament (Figs. 2.13 and 2.16).

There is mention of Greenhill in 1974 stating that "the time of surgical treatment is over" due to the development of radiotherapy. From that time onward, one might wonder if the development of RH techniques also came to a standstill. Indeed, until the 1980s, the shortcomings in Latzko/Okabayashi's RH remained almost ignored.

During the 1980s, the author believed that conventional RH based on classical anatomy is the solution for prevention of intraoperative hemorrhaging and postoperative bladder paralysis.

The author, at that time, was especially interested in the intermediate zone, for it was only depicted as a blank area in Fig. 2.1 by P&A. Both P&A and Reiffenstuhl supported Mackenrodt's description "Fiber bundles extend from the pelvic fascia and attach to the posterior wall of the cervix." However, there was no depiction or mention of visceral vessels even though they must have been aware of their existence within the ligament. In his surgical manual, Reiffenstuhl introduced P&A's connective tissue ground bundle also known as Amreich's connective tissue foundation, Hafferl's intrapelvic body, and Pernkopf's nerve vessel conductor plate. Going away a little from the point, the reason why Reiffenstuhl in 1982 did not follow Pernkopf's view of 1943 illustrated in Fig. 2.14 may be that he, as a scientist, had a strong attachment and faith in P&A's basic anatomy.

The author surmises that the reason why P&A did not depict vessels on Fig. 2.1 was conceivably that observations the surgeons experienced were in conflict with the history/tradition of basic anatomy, causing them distress. Did they, then, entrust to future gynecologists in finding a solution to this intermediate zone being drawn as a vertical blank? The author's response or answer to this query is that it is possible for the longitudinal vessel stumps shown in the author's Fig. 2.13 and vessel arrangement in Fig. 2.20 to be fitted into this blank area (Fig. 3.8). The author personally experienced the result of the differing anatomic views between Pernkopf and Reiffenstuhl (1964, 1982) and what a great impact it has had on development of RH (Figs. 2.18 and 2.21).

In the following paragraphs, the author will demonstrate how he tried to verify his NSRH by fresh cadaver dissection so as to establish preventive measures for intraoperative hemorrhaging and bladder paralysis.

2.2 *Mock Dissection for the Supporting System*

Conforming to RH procedure on a fresh cadaver, the author dissected the supporting system, or *the lateral support consisting of the vesicohypogastric fascia including TCL and the lateral rectal ligament*. From this acquired knowledge and experience, he proceeded to reexamine the L&S/Okabayashi procedures and/or conventional RH, and to construct the anatomic framework for his RH approach, resulting in a) lateral view of the supporting system, b) posterior view of the supporting system, and c) anterior view of the supporting system.

2.2.1 Lateral View of the Supporting System (SS) in a Fresh Cadaver

Figure 3.5 depicts the left SS with the uterus and bladder being pulled cranially to the contralateral side, while the paravesical and pararectal spaces are extensively developed, so that the lateral SS can be observed from a left anterosuperior perspective. As seen in Fig. 3.19, the medial SS has not yet been dissected, and the anterior aspect of the lateral SS is covered by the so-called fascia composed of fatty-areolar connective tissue and a vascular sheath. Intraoperative findings are shown in Fig. 2.20 with the fascia dissected using CUSA, exposing the vessels. Figure 3.5 also shows the separated SS in conventional RH and is represented by a continuum extending from the lateral umbilical artery/ligament to the pelvic floor. Also, in conventional RH, the lateral parametrium, or TCL including the lateral rectal ligament, is clamped and excised en bloc with the areolar connective tissue attached. During such surgery, sliding of ligatures from SS is experienced, leading to a risk of massive hemorrhage, as illustrated in Figs. 2.8 and 2.18.

The glossy membrane covering the pelvic floor in Fig. 3.5 corresponds to the superior fascia of the levator ani. Mackenrodt referred to this fascia as the inferior continuation of TCL, or short fibrous bundle. As depicted in Pernkopf's illustration (Fig. 2.14), SS corresponds to a neurovascular bundle covered by fascia. Therefore, the short fibrous bundle, which is a fascia, connects only to the anterior fascia of SS. P&A removed both SS and the short fibrous bundle simultaneously (panel (**b**) of Fig. 2.4).

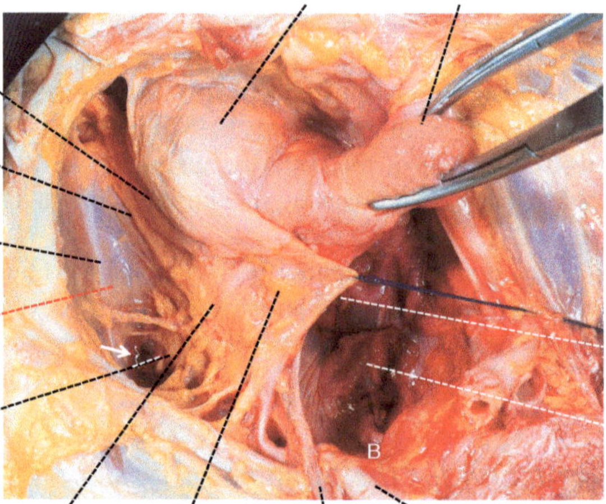

Fig. 3.5 The supporting system and paravesical space
This photograph is of an anatomic dissection on a fresh cadaver. It shows the developed left paravesical space, elevating the clamped uterus with forceps, and the lateral umbilical ligament being pulled superiorly with a thread. The vesicohypogastric fascia originating from the lateral umbilical ligament together with TCL and the lateral rectal ligament form a continuum, or *SS*. The paravesical space and its superior fascia of the levator ani muscle are developed caudally, connecting to the paracolpium through the tendinous arch of the pelvic fascia. A hole (white arrow) has been created in the transition area between SS, or P&A's frontal connective tissue ground bundle, and superior levator fascia, or P&A's horizontal connective tissue ground bundle, to allow entry into the lower portion of the pararectal space. (Reproduced from Yabuki et al. 2005)

It can be said P&A regarded the lateral parametrium and paracolpium as having the same tissue morphology, and this can be looked upon as the largest error made by them.

Figure 3.6 is a schematic illustration from a cranial perspective summarizing Figs. 3.5 and Figs. 2.13 to 2.20, illustrating that SS corresponds to the neurovascular bundle that perpendicularly connects the pelvic organs to the pelvic wall.

2.2.2 Posterior View of the Supporting System (SS) in a Fresh Cadaver

Figure 3.7 demonstrates the posterior aspect of SS and Latzko pararectal space developed by caudal traction of the lateral umbilical artery/ligament shown in Fig. 3.5. It shows where the space is exposed from the lateral umbilical ligament/vesicohypogastric fascia to the fascia of the piriformis muscle. It also shows excision of the posterior fascia of SS, preserving the anterior fascia to which visceral branches of the anterior trunks of the internal iliac vessels attach. In addition, the location of the forceps inserted between the ureter and inferior hypogastric nerve plexus indicates the Okabayashi pararectal space, which is an artificial space and excavated between the posterior mesoureter and fascia lining the posterior leaf of the uterine broad ligament.

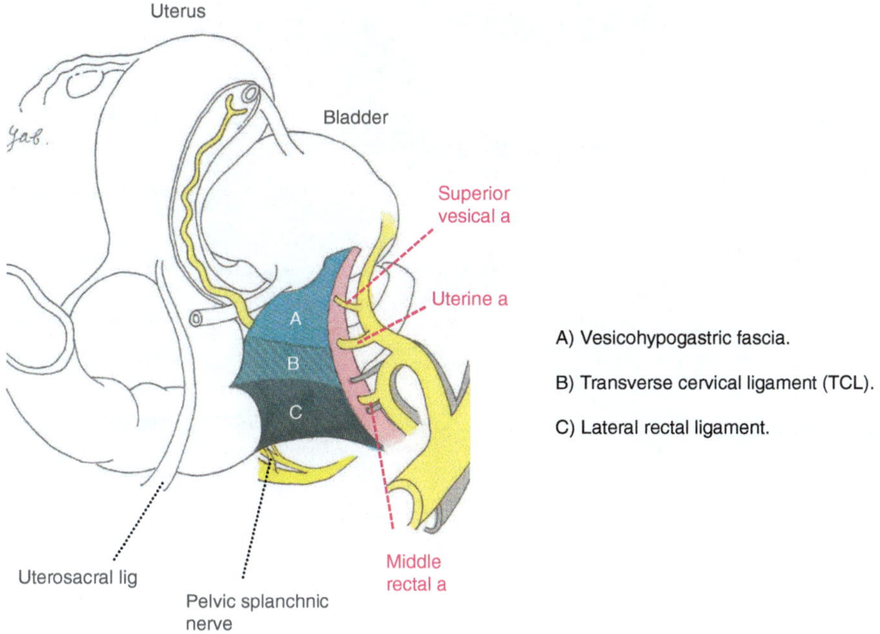

Fig. 3.6 Schematic illustration of the supporting system
Seen from a cranial aspect. The SS consists of the vesicohypogastric fascia, or lamina ligamenti umbilicalis, TCL, and lateral rectal ligament. It forms a single sheet of lamina connecting the pelvic organs, including the bladder, uterus, and rectum, to the pelvic sidewall. One can understand the unnatural appearance of Fig. 3.4 from this schematic illustration in Fig. 3.6. (Reproduced from Yabuki et al. 1996)

Here also in Fig. 3.7, the anterior trunks of the internal iliac vessels are seen dissected and descend almost perpendicularly toward S2–3. While descending, they branch/merge with the visceral branches to/from the umbilical artery leading to the bladder, uterine artery, and superficial and deep uterine veins, which lead to the uterus, inferior vesical artery and vein to the bladder, and visceral branches of the middle rectal artery and vein to the rectum. The intraoperative findings of these separated vessels are seen in Fig. 2.20. The ligaments to which the visceral branches bifurcating from the anterior trunks of the internal iliac vessels belong are the vesicohypogastric fascia, TCL, and lateral rectal ligament. The absence of a named route for the inferior vesical artery and vein may be because, as can be inferred from Fig. 2.1, an alternative route was assumed. Conventional RH involves the en bloc removal of the uterine artery to the middle rectal vessels as shown in Fig. 3.6.

On a fixed cadaver in panel (**a**) of Fig. 3.8 are depicted the stumps of SS dissected in the same manner as during actual surgery, with a histological tissue specimen of SS in panel (**b**). This specimen demonstrates that the lateral ligaments of the bladder, uterus, and rectum surgically form a single plate.

Also seen in Fig. 3.8 is the visceral endopelvic fascia covering the visceral branches of the anterior trunks of the internal iliac vessels that could not be completely dissected. However, no fascia was detected dividing the vesicohypogastric

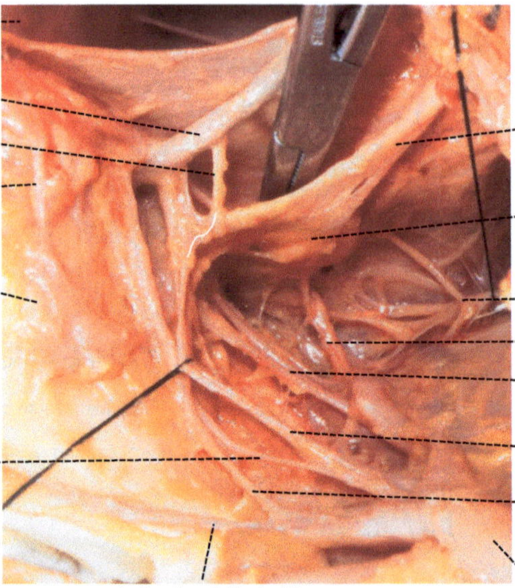

Fig. 3.7 Developed pararectal space on a fresh cadaver
This photograph represents the posterior, or *cranial*, aspect of Fig. 3.5. It shows a view from the aspect of the sacral promontory, depicting a widely developed Latzko's pararectal space with the preservation of the anterior fascia and intraligamentous vessels with only the posterior fascia having been excised to reveal SS. The paravesical space is filled with paper-mâché, exerting tension on SS. The dissected SS forms a single plate from the lateral umbilical ligament to the lateral rectal ligament or sacral aspect. The plate is a continuum of the vesicohypogastric fascia, TCL, and lateral rectal ligament. The visceral terminus of the plate intersects with the pelvic autonomic nerves. The deep uterine vein and S3 pelvic visceral nerve are seen each being pulled with a black thread. The location where the forceps are seen inserted is Okabayashi's pararectal space. (Reproduced from Yabuki et al. 2005)

fascia, TCL, and the lateral rectal ligament. Based on the visceral branches bifurcating from the anterior trunks of the internal iliac vessels in panel (**a**), it can be inferred that the three independent ligaments had already been dissected by the basic anatomic method as shown in Figs. 2.1 and 2.2 and cannot be detected in the area of SS. As suggested by Figs. 2.12 and 2.18, the vessels almost perpendicularly arranged in a row in panels (**a**) and (**b**) of Fig. 3.8 can likely be fitted into the area that P&A referred to as the intermediate zone in Fig. 2.1.

In general, there is little interest during RH procedure in the pathway of the internal iliac artery beyond the branching of the umbilical artery. Figure 3.9 represents a schematic illustration of the anterior trunks of the internal iliac vessels with their visceral branches depicted in Figs. 3.7 and 3.8.

From the anterior trunk of the internal iliac artery, the umbilical artery branches off first. The anterior trunks of the internal iliac artery and vein then proceed in a sacral direction to terminate in the inferior gluteal vessels. Along their course, each of the trunks branches off to (or receives from) the uterine artery and vein, deep uterine vein, inferior vesical artery and vein, and middle rectal artery and vein to/from their respective organs. Furthermore, the bifurcated internal pudendal artery and vein exit the pelvic cavity together with the pudendal nerve through the space

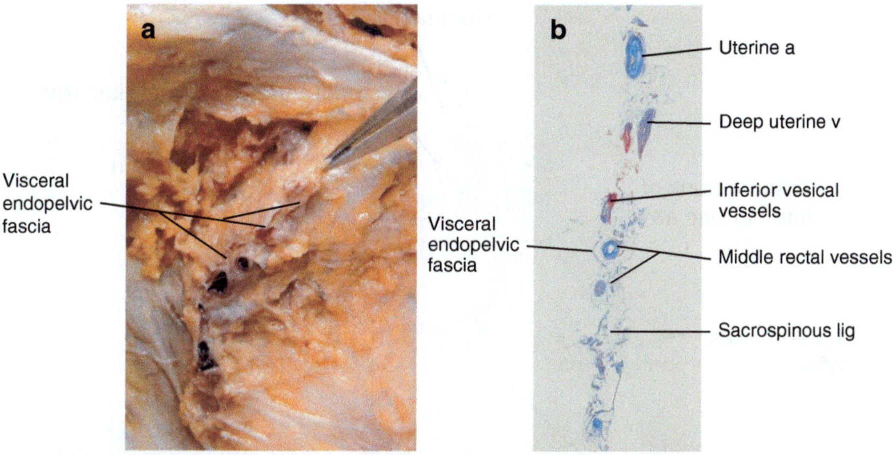

Fig. 3.8 Cross section of the suspensory system and a histological image
Panel (**a**) represents the stumps of the excised bundle between the excavated paravesical and pararectal spaces. The bundle has been separated and severed in a direction perpendicular, rather than in parallel, to the genitalia. Vessels covered with fascia can be observed
Panel (**b**) is a histological image with Elastica van Gieson staining of the stumps of the bundle. The cross section of the blood vessels is arranged longitudinally within the connective tissue. Fascia can be observed, although it is fragmentary. (Reproduced from Yabuki et al. 1991)

underneath the piriformis muscle. The inferior gluteal vessels, the largest terminal branches of the anterior trunk, exit the pelvic cavity after passing through the space between the anterior branches of S2 to S3 from the sacral plexus. The formation of SS is facilitated by branching vessels along the course of the anterior trunks. Pelvic veins accompany all branches of the internal iliac artery except for the umbilical and iliolumbar arteries. In addition, veins from the bladder merge into the deep uterine vein, middle rectal vein, and internal iliac vein to form the vesical drainage system (aa, bb, and cc) (Figs. 3.9 and 3.22). The plate formed by vessels a, b, c, and d in the diagram represents SS (brown rectangle).

Coming back to the hypogastric and pelvic splanchnic nerves depicted in Fig. 3.8, they form the inferior hypogastric plexus, with the sacral splanchnic nerves not yet dissected. When the pararectal space is developed, the relationship between the nerves and visceral vessels becomes almost perpendicular. The middle rectal artery and vein perforate through the center of the inferior hypogastric plexus, while the deep uterine vein passes over the upper margin of the nerve plexus. In conventional RH, the removal of the lateral rectal ligament frequently entails the simultaneous removal of the inferior hypogastric plexus. While some literature suggests that TCL comprises vascular and nervous components (Kobayashi 1961), Fig. 3.7 shows that these components are almost in a craniocaudal relationship.

Figure 3.10 depicts condition of the pelvic sidewall following completion of RH. However, the camera did not capture the course of the internal iliac artery from the bladder region.

In literature on RH, there is often little interest shown in the course of the internal iliac artery and vein after branching from the umbilical artery, resulting in the fact that the visceral branches of the anterior trunks of these internal iliac vessels

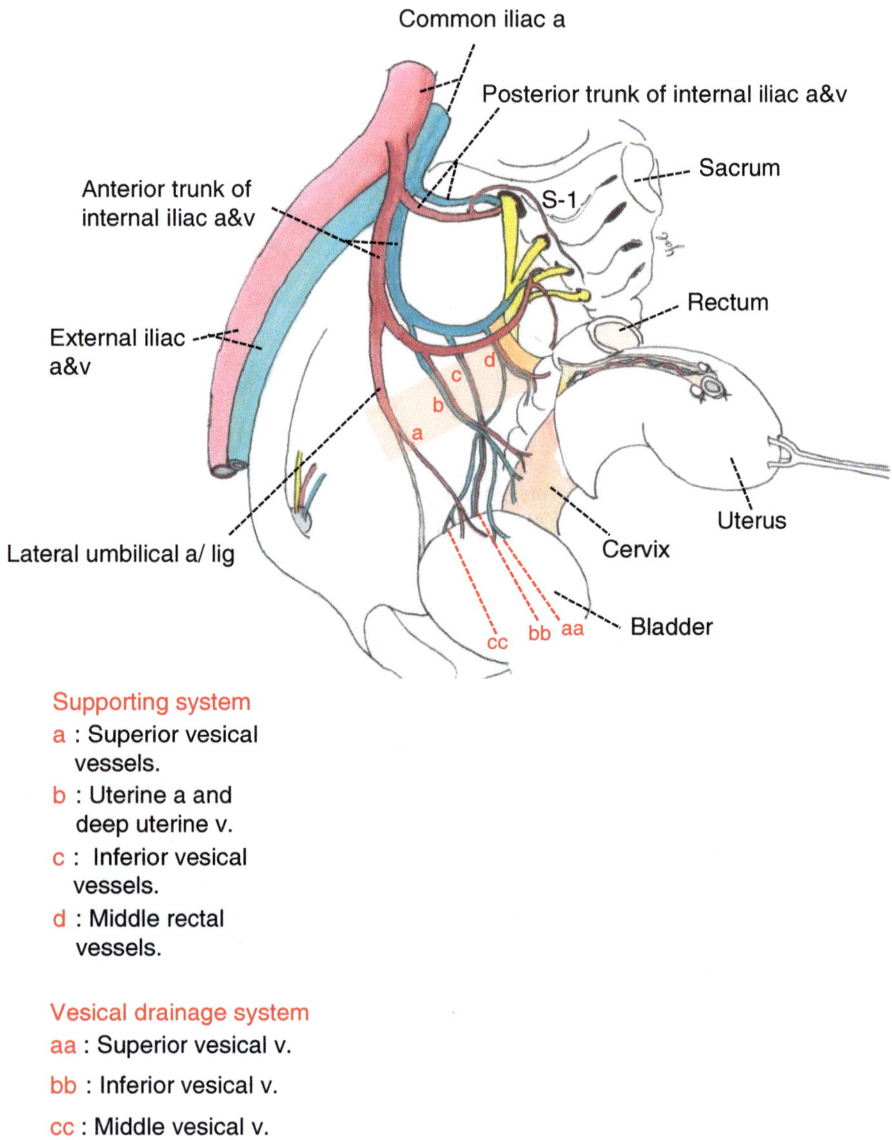

Fig. 3.9 Branches of the anterior trunks of the internal iliac vessels
Pelvic veins follow the course of all branches of the internal iliac artery except for the umbilical and iliolumbar arteries. The anterior trunk of the internal iliac artery first branches off to the umbilical artery. They, then, proceed posteriorly to become the inferior gluteal vessels. During their course, they branch into the uterine artery/vein, deep uterine vein, inferior vesical artery/vein, and middle rectal artery/vein to their respective organs. Furthermore, the branches of the pudendal artery/vein exit the pelvic cavity under the piriformis muscle alongside the pudendal nerve. The inferior gluteal artery/vein is one of the largest terminal branches of the anterior branch and exits the pelvic cavity after passing between the anterior branch of S2 and S3. During the course of the anterior branch, the vessels branching off the uterine artery/vein, deep uterine vein, inferior vesical artery/vein, and middle rectal artery/vein contribute to the formation of SS. In addition, merging with these vessels, veins from the bladder form a drainage system

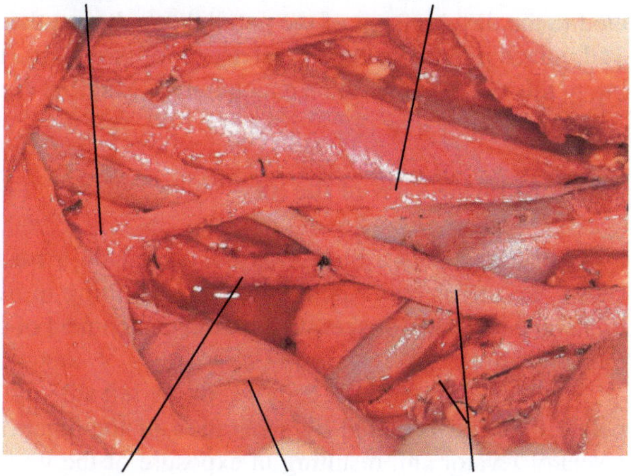

Fig. 3.10 Exposed vessels within the lesser pelvic cavity
Here blood vessels of the right pelvic cavity are shown following completion of pelvic lymphadenectomy with the progression of the anterior trunk of the internal iliac artery obscured by the bladder. In general, the misconception that blood vessels lead toward the coccyx or pubis may be a cause of misunderstandings

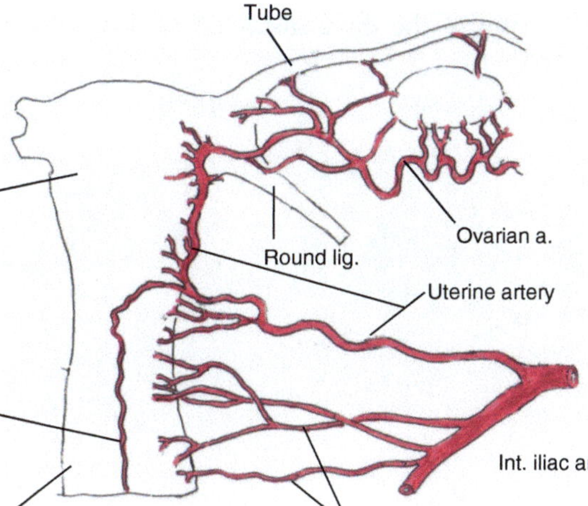

Fig. 3.11 The arteries of the internal organs
This is a description and rough schematic reproduction of Fig. 566 from the 15th edition of Gray's Anatomy: Anatomy; Descriptive and Surgical, 1901, highlighting the arteries. This illustrates that the uterine and vaginal arteries branch independently from the internal iliac artery. The uterine arteries are described in Gray's Anatomy for Students (2005) as follows: "The vaginal artery in women is the equivalent of inferior vesical artery in men and, descending to the vagina, supplies branches to the vagina and to adjacent parts of the bladder and rectum. There is no detailed description of the vaginal vein"

forming SS may go unnoticed. Instead, the internal iliac vessels are repeatedly mistaken as to progress toward the urogenital hiatus.

Figure 3.11 is a diagram taken from the 15th edition of Gray's Anatomy (Pick and Howden 1901), which may give the impression that the uterine and vaginal arteries that branch from the internal iliac artery diverge separately in a pubic direction. This diagrammatic representation in Gray's Anatomy may have contributed to the development of the parallel-attachment theory, which suggests that CL/TCL attach parallel to the lateral aspect of the uterus. Even today, literature adhering to this theory can still be encountered (Magrina et al. 2011).

2.2.3 Anterior View of the SS

Figure 3.12 depicts a dissection conducted on a fresh cadaver. This photograph shows the uterus being pulled upward, resulting in extensive development of the bilateral paravesical spaces with partial detachment of the bladder, revealing SS and the pelvic floor.

On the right side of the cadaver, or the left side of the photograph, is the lateral pelvic ligament revealed by separation of the anterior fascia of SS and superior fascia of levator ani, resulting in exposure of the visceral branches of the anterior trunks of the internal iliac vessels and levator ani muscle. Arranged on a flat plane in Fig. 3.12 are the uterine artery, deep uterine vein, inferior vesical vessels, and middle rectal vessel of the three dissected organs. This finding verifies that the

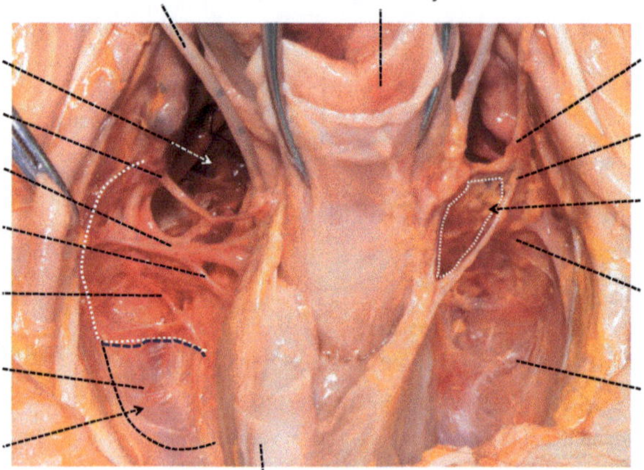

Fig. 3.12 Anterior view of the uterus, vagina, and bladder, with their lateral ligament
This shows an anterior view of the uterus and a partially stripped bladder following an anatomic dissection of a donated 76-year-old fresh cadaver. The uterus has been lifted up, and the paravesical space has been extensively developed. On the left side of the cadaver (right side in the photograph), only the membranous part of the vesicohypogastric fascia, outlined with a white dotted line, has been removed so as to allow this fascia to be folded back and conceal only a portion of TCL. The fasciae of TCL and lateral rectal ligament, and superior fascia of the pelvic diaphragm can now be seen exposed. On the right side of the cadaver (left side in the photograph), the anterior/posterior fasciae of TCL, anterior fascia of the lateral rectal ligament, and superior fascia of the pelvic diaphragm have been excised, thereby exposing the anterior trunks of the internal iliac vessels and levator ani muscle. In this photograph, the visceral branches are seen anastomosed or interconnected, making the identification of the deep uterine vein difficult, but, if this occurs in actual surgery, caution is required. (Reproduced from Yabuki 2023)

relationship between SS and the organs is almost perpendicular, not horizontal. If one synthesizes the findings obtained from Figs. 3.5, 3.7, and 3.12, the relationship between the uterine cervix and TCL is concluded to be perpendicular.

The visceral vessels, or mainly veins, in this cadaver in Fig. 3.12 exhibit complex patterns of fusion and branching, making it difficult to accurately identify them by name. Similar challenges are also encountered in actual surgeries. In addition, locating the middle rectal vessels can be challenging, but confirmation from the pararectal space is relatively straightforward as shown in Fig. 3.7.

The lateral parametrium targeted for resection in the Latzko, Okabayashi, and Meigs procedures encompasses the area from the uterine artery to the middle rectal vessels (dashed white area). This traditional surgical approach was upheld until the end of the twentieth century (Fig. 2.8).

The area indicated by the black dashed line in Fig. 3.12 represents the levator ani muscle. In the Latzko procedure, parametrectomy and paracolpectomy are carried out along the white and black dashed lines drawn along the pelvic sidewall. In contrast, in the Okabayashi RH, parametrectomy (Fig. 2.30) involves the area within the white dashed line, while paracolpectomy involves only the area medial to the tendinous arch of the pelvic fascia as shown in Fig. 3.5. Further details on this will be discussed in the section on the paracolpium (pp. 83–85).

Next, the findings of SS on the left side of the cadaver, or *the right side in the photograph*, are shown in Fig. 3.12. The anterior fascia of SS is seen preserved including the superior fascia of the levator ani except for the vesicohypogastric fascia enclosed by the white dashed line, which has been excised allowing visualization of TCL. In conventional RH, the lateral parametrium, or TCL including the lateral rectal ligament, is removed while the fascia remains attached as it is.

From the findings demonstrated in Figs. 3.5, 3.7, and 3.12, it was concluded that the relationship between TCL and uterine cervix was perpendicular, but to the naked eye, the relationship between the paracolpium and vagina appears horizontal, which is described and verified histologically in the section on the Paracolpium. There is no doubt about the uterine broad ligament attaching parallel to the lateral aspect of the uterus. Moreover, introduction of "the condensation in the base of the broad ligament" of Savage (Fig. 2.11) demonstrated the relationship between CL and uterus as being horizontal (Fig. 2.1).

Historically and traditionally, the relationship among the uterine broad ligament, CL, and paracolpium is believed to be horizontal. In contrast, the author has emphasized that the relationship between the uterus and TCL is perpendicular. It is easy to imagine that an intricate anatomic structure must exist for these three organs that have a totally different morphology being held in the lesser pelvic cavity without hindrance to the function of each organ. The author believes in the existence of at least two bundles in the subperitoneal structure of the lesser pelvic cavity: the longitudinal and transversal bundles. Details on this will be described toward the end of this chapter.

The "Ligament-denial theory" about TCL has existed since the 1930s. Goff (1931), Koster (1933), Berglass and Rubin (1953), Range and Woodburne (1964), Bastian and Lassau (1982), and Fritsch et al. (1992) concluded TCL as "the absence of ligamentous structures". Furthermore, Range stated: "This ligament contained only loose areolar connective tissue enclosing blood vessels, nerves, and lymphatic tissue." Indeed, visceral fascia cannot be defined as far as panels (**b**) of Fig. 2.17 and/or Fig. 2.27 are concerned, but it has been identified in fragments shown in Fig. 3.8. Men are supposed to have Denonvilliers' fascia lying between the rectum and prostate gland, but the corresponding fascia in women is the rectovaginal septum. Indeed, there is a feeling of slight resistance when removing the bladder, although it is difficult to identify it with the naked eye.

3 Clinical Anatomy of the Anterior and Posterior Supports

3.1 Overview

Mackenrodt observed in the fetus that "These fiber bundles, of the same histologic composition as the transverse cervical ligament, are arranged at its upper edge into a rather stringlike band, the uterosacral ligament." He also stated, "At the level of the internal os still other fibrous processes extend from the transverse ligament, past the lateral wall of the bladder, and anterior to the part of the pelvic fascia that extends from the arcus tendinous to the posterior wall of the symphysis: the pubo-vesico-uterine ligament." These findings suggest that a portion of the TCL fascia reflects craniocaudally on the uterus, connecting to the uterosacral pubo-vesico-uterine ligaments. TCL, as we know it, is simply not only a fibrous bundle but also functions as a pathway for blood vessels (Fig. 3.9). Moreover, the existence of a neurovascular bundle, or *mesoureter*, is also recognized (Figs. 3.1, 3.2, and 3.3). Savage/Kocks refers to CL as a bundle that connects the uterine cervix and mesoureter, but this should be distinguished from TCL.

In the following section, the author arranges the vesicouterine ligament and anterior mesoureter into the anterior support and the posterior mesoureter into the posterior support together with an anatomic examination of these two supporting systems. The surgical procedure for the anterior/posterior supports of Latzko and Okabayashi has already been described. The author expects readers to associate the following surgical procedures with anatomy.

Panel (**a**) is a horizontal section through the lateral umbilical ligament and upper aspect of TCL
Panel (**b**): Horizontally sectioned tissue at the level of the ureter. The width of the specimen from the medial aspect of the ureter to the lateral aspect of the uterine cervix is 7 mm with approximately 30% reduction
Panel (**c**) is a horizontal section centered on the inferior hypogastric plexus
The dashed ellipse regions marked on the 3 tissue samples depicted in panels (**a**), (**b**), and (**c**) represent a cylinder filled with loose connective tissue but few blood vessels. The author has named the space excavated within the dashed ellipse region of panel (**a**) as the "fourth space." (Reproduced from Yabuki 2016)

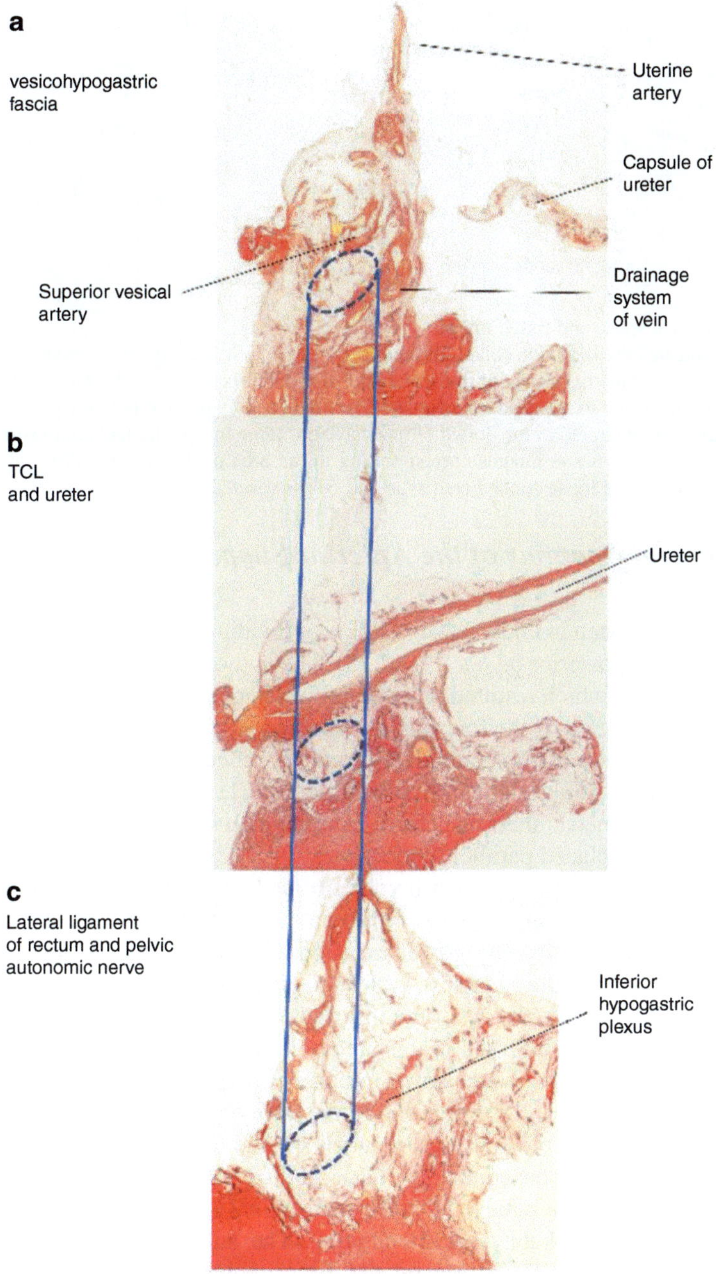

Fig. 3.13 Horizontal section of the supporting system
The pelvic organs and their lateral tissues were removed during cadaver dissection and a stent was inserted parallel to the ureter, followed by fixation in formalin. Three horizontally sectioned tissue specimens with Elastica van Gieson staining were obtained and are demonstrated in panels (**a**), (**b**), and (**c**)

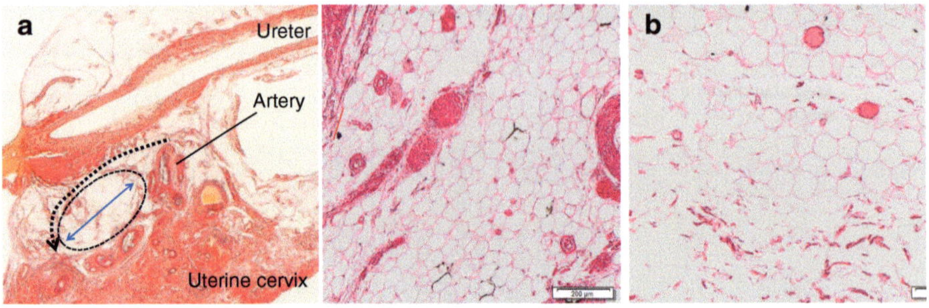

Fig. 3.14 Fourth space and tissue image
Panel (**a**) indicates the direction (black dashed arrow) in which Okabayshi's paravaginal space is excavated along the medial aspect of the ureter and, also the direction (blue double arrow) in which the author's "open-pit" excavation is carried out. It can be concluded that both the paravaginal and fourth spaces demonstrated in the dotted ellipse have the same morphological composition
Panel (**b**) depicts two tissue images corresponding to the area of the dashed ellipse in panel (**a**) filled with adipose and loose connective tissue and is less vascular

3.2 Clinical Anatomy of the Anterior Support

The anterior approach in Okabayashi's RH is of dividing the vesicouterine ligament into anterior and posterior layers (Fig. 2.25). The author examined these two layers histoanatomically, which resulted in a new proposed concept and surgical approach, namely, the excavation of the fourth space and nerve-sparing surgery.

Figure 3.13 shows histopathological tissue specimens from three dissected pelvic viscera, that is, the vesicohypogastric fascia, TCL, and lateral rectal ligament, horizontally sectioned at their respective levels, which were previously fixed in formalin with a stent placed parallel to the ureter.

Okabayashi's anterior approach involves tunneling with forceps inserted along the medial aspect of the ureter in the direction of the black curved dashed arrow in panel (**a**) of Fig. 3.14, repeating roof excision and ligature two to three times. A drawback of this procedure is the risk of damaging the ureter and/or blood vessels due to the inability to see the tip of the inserted forceps.

However, the tissue observed in this area by the author consisted of adipose tissue and loose connective tissue shown in panel (**b**). This tissue morphology is the same as that for the area corresponding to the vesicohypogastric fascia and lateral rectal ligament (dashed blue ellipses in panels (**a**) and (**c**) of Fig. 3.13) and assumed to be a cylinder of areolar connective tissue indicated in Fig. 3.13. Based on this tissue finding, the author believed that the paravaginal space could be directly excavated without using Okabayashi's technique. The author executed this method, called "open-pit mining," and named the space thus created the "fourth space." (Yabuki et al. 1996) This term denotes a fourth space following the paravesical, Latzko's pararectal, and Okabayashi's pararectal spaces (Fig. 3.15).

The excavation site of the fourth space is the region of fatty areolar connective tissue between the vesicouterine ligament, also known as the pubocervical ligament, or bladder pillar, and ureter (Fig. 3.15). This excavation method is described in the Chapter on Surgical Procedures. After excavating the fourth space, the bladder pillar is excised.

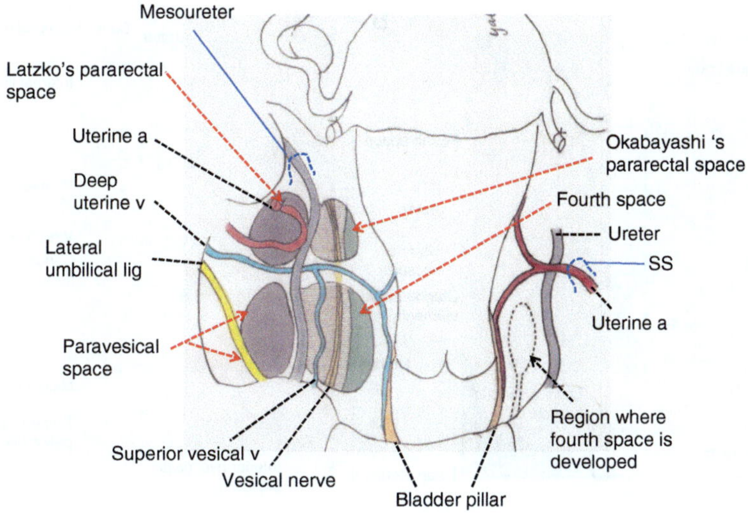

Fig. 3.15 Artificial fascial compartment for RH
This illustration shows the markings of the uterine artery/vein and ureter used as reference points in RH for excavation of the four spaces, resulting in SS and mesoureter being dissected. The anterior mesoureter, which is freed between the paravesical and fourth spaces, contains the vesical nerve branches from the inferior hypogastric plexus and vesical vessels connecting SS to the bladder. (Reproduced from Yabuki 2020)

The lamina hanging down from the ureter, which is sandwiched between the fourth and paravesical spaces, corresponds to either Okabayashi's posterior layer or the author's anterior mesoureter. Figure 3.16 depicts a perpendicular, or frontal, section of the pelvic organs along the cylindrical region of the tissues shown in Fig. 3.13.

Figure 3.16 shows a frontal section of the transitional area between the uterine body and uterine cervix. Panel (**a**) shows a macroscopic tissue dissection, and panel (**b**) shows a microscopic tissue sample taken from a detail window in panel (**a**). The portion sandwiched between the two red dashed lines in panel (**a**) is the lateral rectal ligament within which a cross section of the middle rectal vessels is visible. The middle rectal vessels pass through the inferior hypogastric plexus and traverse the lateral rectal ligament to reach the rectum. Panel (**b**) shows where TCL attaches to the uterine cervix on a line formed by the stumps of the deep uterine vein and uterine artery. The stumps labeled with a's representing the uterine artery near to the internal iliac artery are considered to be the approximate origin of TCL. The area connecting these points represents TCL. It is suggested that TCL and the lateral rectal ligament form a continuous plane perpendicular to the organs. Figure 3.17 shows a view from the lateral aspect of the lesser pelvic cavity with the uterus pulled cranially following the excavation of the paravesical and pararectal spaces in a fresh cadaver.

The artificial manipulation in Fig. 3.17 cannot be perfectly compared with Fig. 3.16, but from these two figures, it is evident that the positional relationships of the hypogastric nerve, pelvic splanchnic nerves, inferior hypogastric plexus, and visceral nerve can be observed. It is also apparent that the visceral nerve reaches the bladder from the inferior hypogastric plexus at a steep angle and distributes widely.

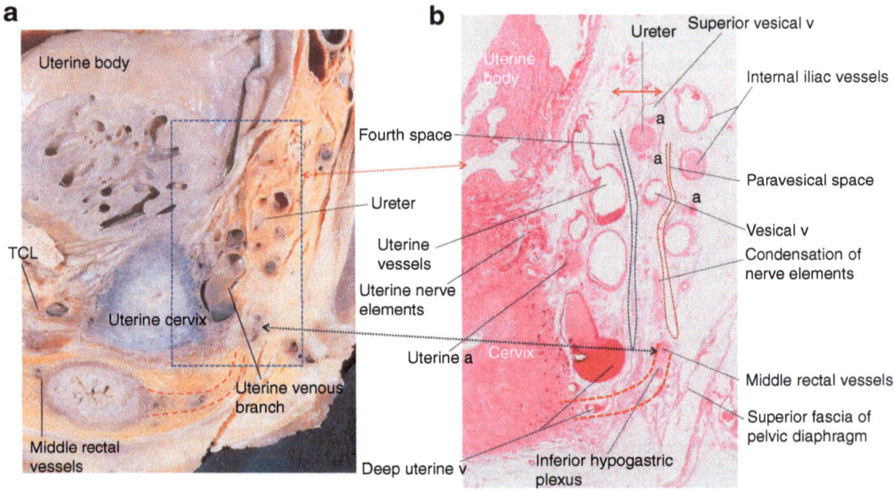

Fig. 3.16 Macroscopic and histological images of the area around the uterine isthmus
Panel (**a**) depicts a macroscopic sliced tissue specimen taken from a 90-year-old female donor at the corpocervical junction of the uterus, which lies between the uterine body and cervix. There is some slight lateral displacement in this cross-sectional view. (Reproduced from Yabuki et al. 2011)
Panel (**b**) depicts a perpendicularly sectioned tissue specimen of the lateral parametrium. This histological section with hematoxylin and eosin tissue staining was taken from the dashed rectangular area in panel (**a**). The tissue connecting the stumps of the uterine artery and deep uterine vein, as well as the stump of the internal iliac artery/vein, corresponds to TCL. The lateral rectal ligament exists in the region sandwiched between the two dashed red lines connecting the middle rectal vessels, which penetrate the inferior hypogastric plexus, and vessels alongside the rectum. This observation suggests that TCL and the lateral rectal ligament form a continuum. The nerve elements seen extending linearly from the inferior hypogastric plexus to the bladder are the vesical branches of the autonomic nerve

In panel (**b**) of Fig. 3.16, the area of loose connective tissue between the internal iliac vessels and vesicouterine vascular plexus (two red arrows) represents the lesser pelvic cavity. This cavity is divided into medial and lateral compartments by a lamina consisting of (a) the vesical autonomic nerve branch extending from the inferior hypogastric plexus to the ureter and (b) vessels from the bladder. The inferior hypogastric plexus contains many myelinated nerve fibers, while unmyelinated nerve fibers are predominantly observed around the uterine cervix (Niikura et al. 2007). In the compartment medial to the autonomic nerve, there is an area filled with fatty-areolar connective tissue sandwiched between the visceral endopelvic fascia and nerve elements. The fossa excavated in this area is the fourth space (blue dashed line). In the compartment lateral to the autonomic nerve, there is an area filled with fatty-areolar connective tissue sandwiched between the parietal endopelvic fascia and nerve elements, namely, the retroperitoneal space. The space excavated here is the paravesical space (brown dashed line in panel (**b**) of Fig. 3.16). From these findings, it can be concluded that the anterior mesoureter is created between the fourth and paravesical spaces, which is a neurovascular bundle descending from the ureter. The reason the author assigned the name "anterior mesoureter" is because Okabayashi's anatomic definition of the posterior layer was ambiguous.

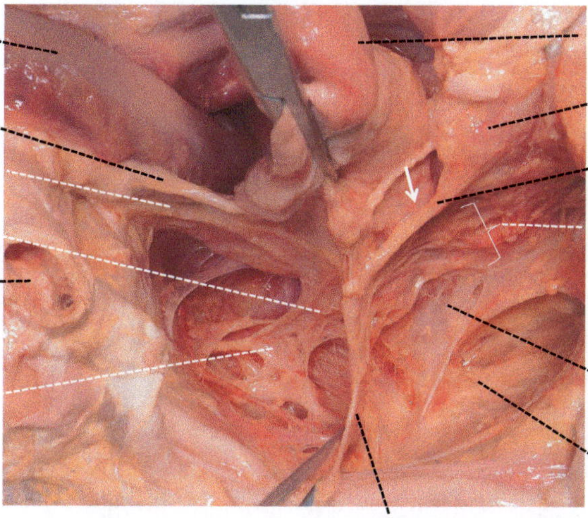

Fig. 3.17 Developed pelvic cavity and pelvic nerves
This photograph taken from a bird's-eye-view shows an anatomic dissection on a fresh cadaver with the pelvic visceral peritoneum having been removed. The paravesical and Latzko's pararectal spaces are seen developed, exposing SS between the two spaces. The pelvic visceral nerves from S2 to S4 are separated in the pararectal space. In the paravesical space, a portion of the superior levator fascia has been removed, exposing the levator ani muscle. The inferior hypogastric plexus is formed by the hypogastric nerve and pelvic/sacral splanchnic nerves. The vesical nerve branches with the vesical vein running alongside are distributed to the bladder (Fig. 3.21). (Reproduced from Yabuki et al. 2005)

Based on these findings, the author classified the anterior support into three components: (a) the true fascial ligament connecting the bladder and uterus, known as the vesicouterine ligament or bladder pillar; (b) the area of areolar connective tissue where the fourth space is excavated between the bladder pillar and ureter; and c) the neurovascular bundle, or *anterior mesoureter*, hanging from the ureter. Each of these components possesses an independent function in connecting the bladder and uterus/TCL.

An attempt was made to elucidate the anatomic relationship between the vesical nerve branch and vascular branches passing along the anterior mesoureter. The vesical nerve branch emerging from the inferior hypogastric plexus seen in panel (**c**) of Figs. 3.13 or 3.17 reaches the posterior aspect of the ureter at a sharp angle as depicted in Fig. 3.17. While the trajectory of the ureter curves medially, the nerve branch reaches the bladder almost perpendicularly (panels (**b**) of Figs. 2.17 and 3.17). The vessels within the anterior mesoureter depicted in panel (**b**) of Fig. 3.17 can always be observed even in surgical specimens as demonstrated by the superior vesical vein in Fig. 4.30.

Figure 3.18 illustrates a state where the uterus in Fig. 3.12 is seen strongly pulled to the left.

Figures 3.12 and 3.18 infer that the ureter passes under the uterine artery and connects to the bladder, and the hypogastric nerve passes alongside the dorsal aspect of the ureter and connects to the inferior hypogastric plexus (Fig. 3.21). Also,

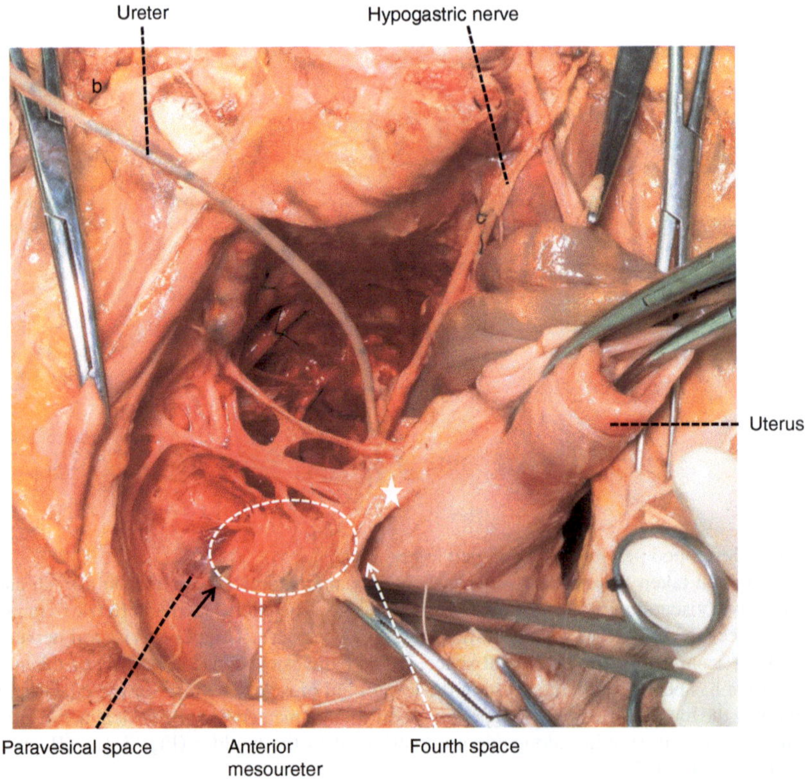

Fig. 3.18 Excavation of the fourth space and separated anterior mesoureter
This is a photograph showing a simulated dissection on a fresh cadaver for RH. The uterus is being pulled to the left, exposing the right SS. Metzenbaum scissors are seen inserted between the ureter and uterine cervix to excavate the fourth space. The tip of the scissors (black arrow) is seen at the pelvic floor. The dashed white ellipse represents the anterior mesoureter, and the space between the back of the scissors and uterine cervix is the fourth space. (Reproduced from Yabuki et al. 2005)

Fig. 3.18 depicts the creation of the fourth space by the insertion of scissors between the uterine cervix and ureter, extending the tips into the paravesical space. A white arrow indicates the insertion point of the scissors in Fig. 3.17. It is conjectured that a portion of the vascular branches of SS reflects anteriorly along the course of the ureter and hypogastric nerve, forming the anterior mesoureter (dashed white ellipse in Fig. 3.18). The anterior mesoureter is dissected between the fourth and paravesical spaces shown in a fresh cadaver in Fig. 3.19.

The hypogastric nerve in this figure enters the inferior hypogastric plexus at a point where the mesoureter and SS intersect, and the nerve branches bifurcating from the nerve plexus pass through the anterior mesoureter and distribute to the bladder. In contrast, a vein, or *the superior vesical vein coined by the author*, from the bladder joins the deep uterine vein. The deep uterine vein runs adjacent to the ventral aspect of the nerve plexus, connecting to the uterine cervix.

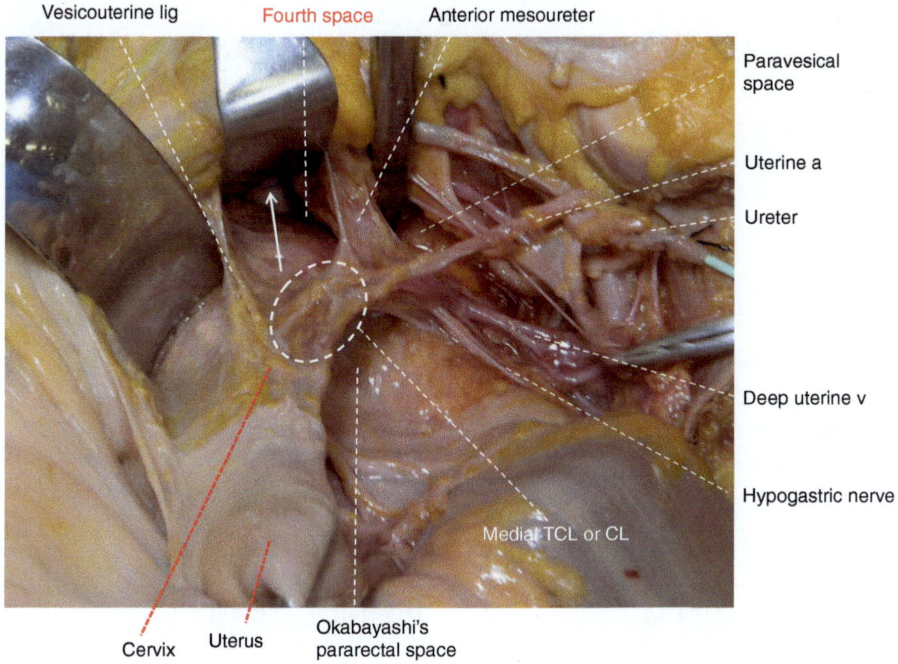

Fig. 3.19 Excavated fourth space and anterior mesoureter
This is an anatomic dissection of a fresh cadaver. The paravesical space, anterior mesoureter, and fourth space are seen aligned. The ureter has been moved to the anterolateral aspect of the cadaver. The area indicated by the dashed white ellipse corresponds to the medial TCL. The fourth space that is excavated within CL is seen extended in a caudal direction (white arrow)

Panel (**a**) of Fig. 3.20 shows a frontally sectioned histological image of the anterior mesoureter. Numerous nerve endings are visible on the dorsal aspect of the superior vesical vein. Panel (**b**) depicts a sagittally sectioned histological image passing through the center of the ureter. Many nerve endings (red circles) are seen present within the nerve branches of the ureter and/or anterior mesoureter.

Figure 3.21 depicts anatomic findings by a skeletonized dissection of the anterior mesoureter. Figures 3.7, 3.9, and 3.20 demonstrate the superior and inferior vesical veins converging from the bladder to the deep uterine vein and internal iliac vein. The vesical nerve branches from the inferior hypogastric plexus are surrounded by the superior and inferior vesical veins and distribute to the bladder. These nerves are part of the vesical nerve branches indicated in Fig. 3.17.

Regarding the lymphatic drainage pathway of the anterior mesoureter, Kraima et al. stated, "No lymph vessels draining the cervix uteri were detected in the vesicouterine ligament," (Curtis et al. 1940) although the author did not go into any detailed investigation of this statement in regard to Figs. 3.20 and 3.21. This information suggests excising only the superior vesical vein within the anterior mesoureter and preserving the deep nerves does not affect metastasis of early cancer of the uterine

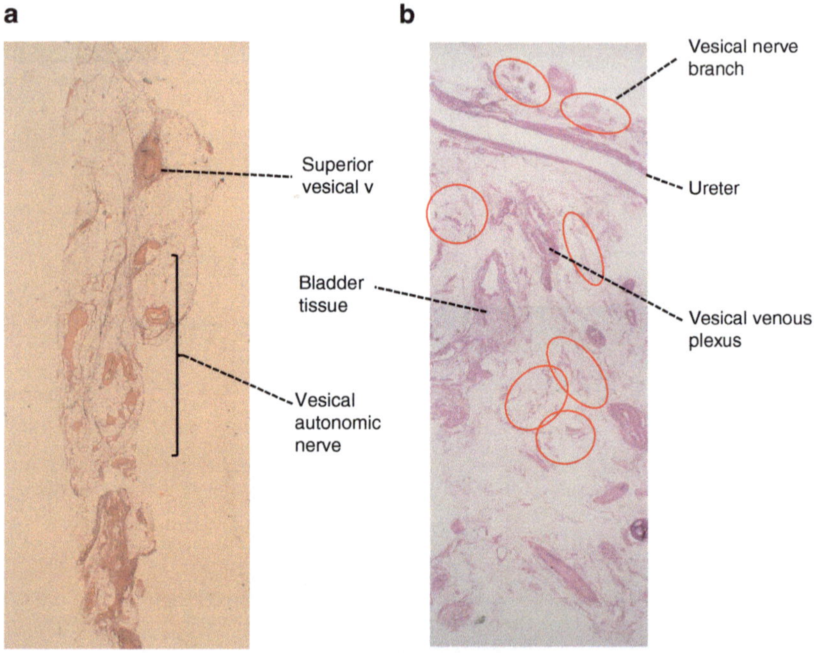

Fig. 3.20 Histological images of the severed anterior mesoureter
Panel (**a**) shows a histological image of transversely sectioned anterior mesoureter tissue depicted in Fig. 3.20 with 2.5 times magnification and Elastica van Gieson staining. This image of the anterior mesoureter appears upon excavation of the fourth space and paravesical space (Fig. 3.18). The vesical nerve branches containing nerve ganglions are concentrated deep within the superior vesical veins. (Reproduced from Yabuki et al. 1996)
Panel (**b**) shows a sagittally sliced histological image of the anterior mesoureter severed along the long axis of the ureter. The left side of the figure represents the caudal aspect, and the areas enclosed by the red ellipses are the vesical nerve branches. Cross sections of the nerves can be widely observed around the ureter and blood vessels. (Reproduced from Yabuki 2016)

cervix. Based on my experience, I propose that cervical cancer with infiltration or metastasis to the posterior layer should be classified as FIGO Stage Three.

Figure 3.22 illustrates three venous branches from the bladder draining into the anterior trunk of the internal iliac vein via the anterior mesoureter and SS. This is demonstrated respectively as follows: The superior vesical vein (Fig. 4.34) via the deep uterine vein; the inferior vesical vein (Fig. 3.7) draining directly; and the middle vesical vein (Fig. 4.43) via the middle rectal vein. The superior and middle vesical veins are the author's own anatomic terms. The superior, inferior, and middle vesical veins together with the deep uterine vein, inferior vesical vein, and middle rectal vein can be surgically arranged into two plate-like structures, seen in gray and light blue in this figure.

According to Gray's Anatomy for Students (Drake et al. 2005), the vaginal artery is said to be equivalent to the inferior vesical artery in men. For the vesical veins, it is only mentioned that they form a vesical plexus of veins.

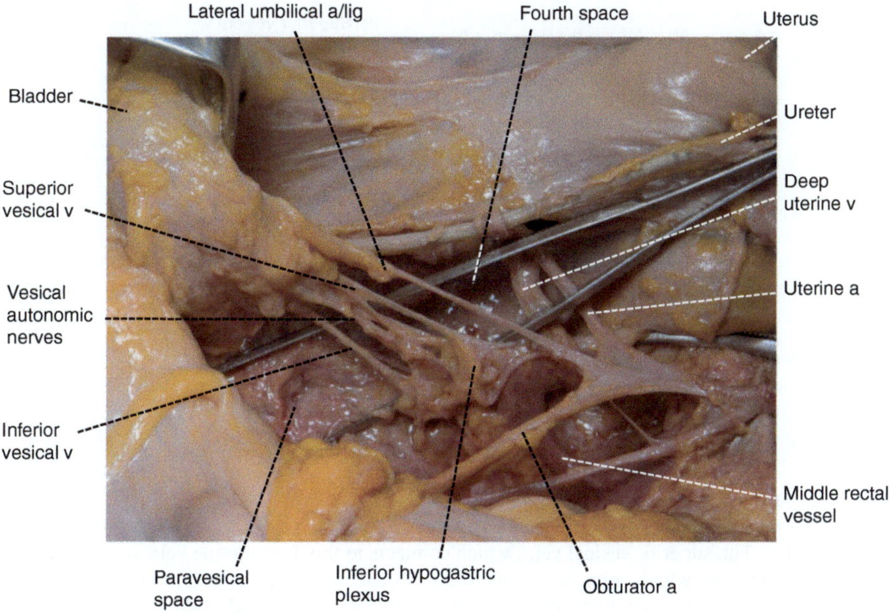

Fig. 3.21 Dissection of the anterior mesoureter on a fresh cadaver
This photograph shows the uterus being strongly pulled in a direction of the promontory and the stripped bladder being pushed with a hook toward the pubis. The pelvic plexus has been detached from the rectovaginal ligament, and the vesical nerve branches of the anterior mesoureter are separated. Simultaneously, the lateral umbilical, uterine, and superior vesical arteries are separated from the internal iliac artery, exposing the superior vesical vein that drains into the deep uterine vein. Also, in this photograph, the lateral umbilical ligament and anterior mesoureter can be seen arranged perpendicularly, but in the living body, the anterior mesoureter is positioned more medially. The fourth space corresponds to the space where the forceps are seen inserted. (Reproduced from Yabuki 2023)

The observed vaginal artery is primarily formed by the descending uterine artery or often branches from the uterine artery. The author has never encountered a case where branches directly bifurcated from the internal iliac artery as depicted in Fig. 3.11. In contrast, the deep uterine vein, also known as the vaginal vein, drains from the uterine vascular branches into the internal iliac vein, as mentioned earlier. These veins become crucial targets for resection in RH. Identifying these veins, which are dilated veins of the bladder or uterus, would indeed be challenging when viewed from the aspect of basic anatomy especially on fixed cadavers. Moreover, this anatomic ambiguity regarding the branching of the deep uterine vein from the vagina might have led to the non-excision of the deep uterine vein in RH carried out by Cibula et al. (2011). The non-resection of the deep uterine vein also entails the non-handling of the anterior mesoureter concurrently. However, calling this surgery RH while leaving a part of TCL intact, or referring to it as nerve-sparing surgery while completely avoiding the nerves, seems overly lenient.

Figure 3.23 is a composite image created on a computer by extracting the vessels and nerves from their surrounding tissue in Figs. 3.7 and 3.21 to enable an

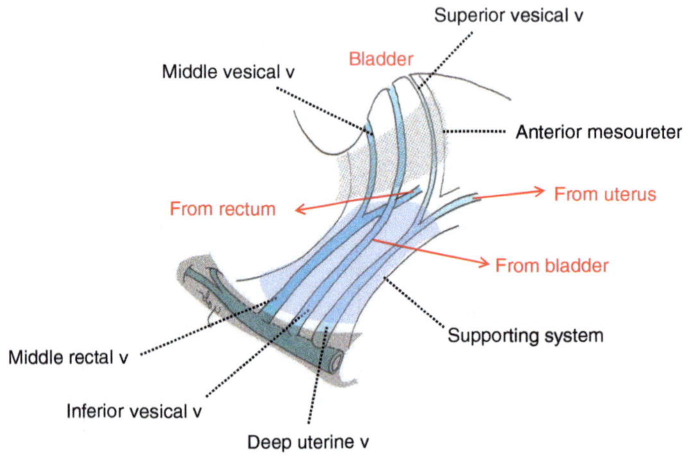

Fig. 3.22 Drainage system of the bladder
The following venous network is referred to by the author as the drainage system, which consists of three veins. The superior vesical vein, which connects to the deep uterine vein and bladder; the inferior vesical vein, which connects to the anterior branch of the internal iliac vein and bladder; and the middle vesical vein, which connects to the middle rectal vein and bladder, all of which pass through the anterior mesoureter. (Reproduced from Yabuki et al. 1996)

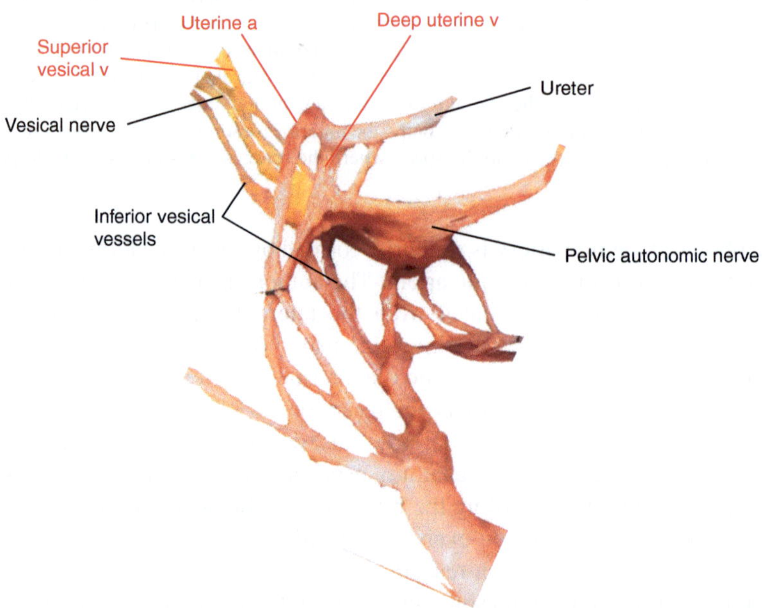

Fig. 3.23 Composite diagram of vessels of the supporting system, and pelvic autonomic nerve
By the removal of SS that acts as a barrier, an attempt was made to create a composite of vessels and nerves from those shown separated in Figs. 3.7 and 3.21. In RH with an emphasis on QOL, excision should take place around the area of the named blood vessels highlighted in red

understanding of the vascular and neural connections between SS and the anterior mesoureter. As a result, the relationship between the nerves and blood vessels during the intraoperative development of the pararectal space is clarified, indicating a craniocaudal rather than a ventrodorsal, or superficial-deep, orientation.

The surgical procedure for sparing bladder function in the 1970s placed emphasis on the preservation of the pelvic splanchnic nerves. The primary reason for this was that, at that time, the lateral rectal ligament was still considered a part of the parametrium and excised, and the pelvic splanchnic nerves, which were anatomically at the same level, were also subject to excision (Fig. 3.17). Therefore, until the author's publication on non-excision of the lateral rectal ligament, neither the inferior hypogastric plexus nor the hypogastric nerve was discussed as a target for preservation. In 2004, Raspagliesi recognized the author as a pioneer of nerve-sparing surgery (Raspagliesi et al. 2004), bringing attention to his nerve-sparing surgery through non-excision of the lateral rectal ligament and preservation of the vesical nerve branches.

Anatomically defining the area known as the paracystium presents a serious challenge. Even P&A's explanation of the ascending and sagittal bladder pillars is ambiguous (Peham and Amreich 1934). The author believes that both the drainage system of the anterior mesoureter and vesicohypogastric fascia of the lateral umbilical artery/ligament form the paracystium (red circle in Fig. 3.24).

Regarding the parametrium, the vascular supply of the reflected TCL divides into the ascending and descending vessels, distributing to the uterus and vagina (Figs. 3.24 and 3.25).

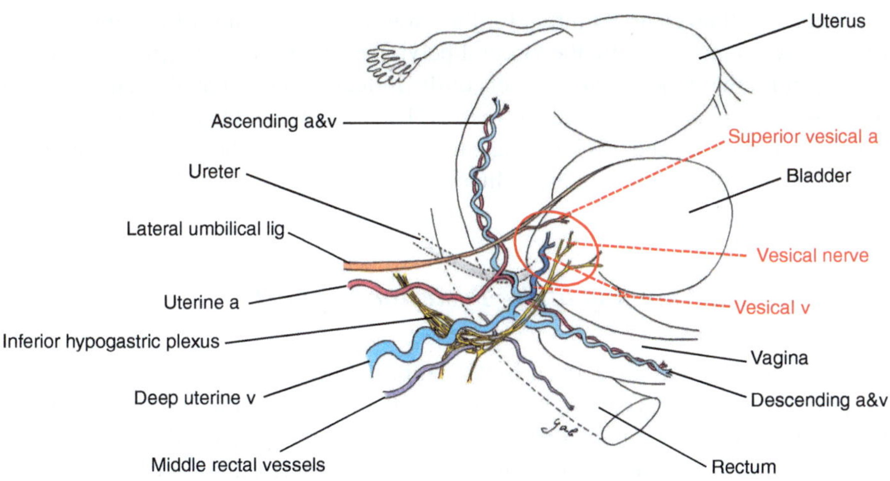

Fig. 3.24 Visceral terminus of vessels of the supporting system and distribution
As seen from a right anterior perspective, this schematic illustration shows the distribution of the blood vessels and vesical nerves to the organs. Depicted with a red circle, the vesical vein and vesical nerve branches are seen passing through the anterior mesoureter with multiple veins represented by a single vein. The blood vessels to the uterus and rectum branch into the ascending and descending branches and distribute to the organs passing through CL and paraproctium

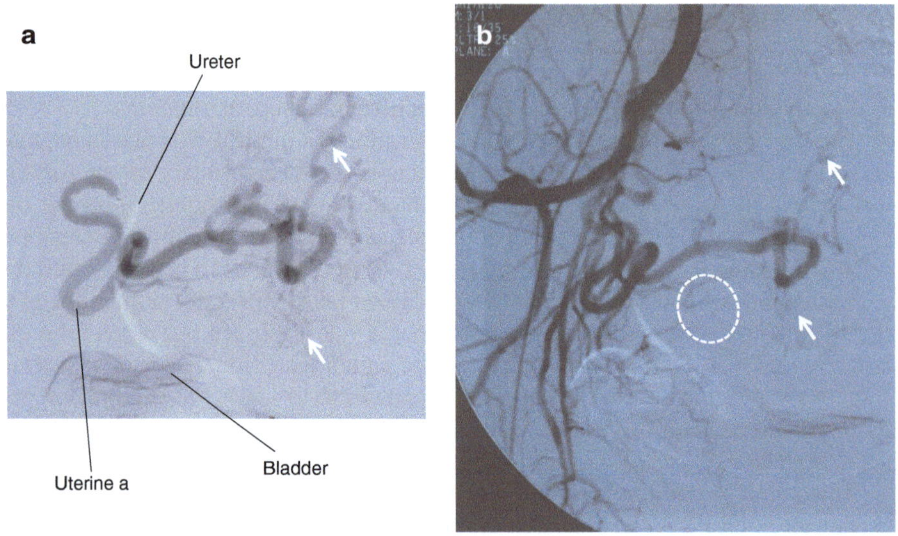

Fig. 3.25 Angiogram of the uterine artery
Panel (**a**): For the purpose of neoadjuvant intra-arterial chemotherapy, a contrast medium was administered into the uterine artery to enable visualization of the ureter with this medium later being excreted in the urine. The uterine artery can be seen meandering in loops before reaching the uterus, and white arrows indicate its ascending and descending branches
Panel (**b**) shows an overall view with the area around the ureterovesical junction being enhanced by a contrast medium. The dashed ellipse indicates an area with poor vascularity, which is presumed to correspond to the fourth space

There is still no clear definition for the paraproctium, but it is often referred to as the mesorectum covered by the visceral pelvic fascia, or *fascia propria*. Within the mesorectum, the middle rectal vessels of the reflected lateral rectal ligament merge with the superior and inferior rectal vessels. The presence of the middle rectal artery is reported to be around 20–90% (Sato and Sato 1991), but there has been no mention of the middle rectal vein in the literature.

3.3 Clinical Anatomy of the Posterior Support

The posterior support envisioned by the author structurally resembles the anterior support. From a medial aspect, it is comprised in the order of the sacro/rectouterine ligament, a true fascial ligament, Okabayashi's pararectal space that is filled with areolar connective tissue, and, finally, the ureter/posterior mesoureter. Beginning with Blatsdell (1917), the uterosacral ligament has been considered as a part of the suspensory mechanism of the uterus, and Bastian et al. (1982) referenced Curtis et al.'s thesis (1940) and stated: "... the uterosacral ligament and paracervix lie in direct continuity with each other together form a common pedicle" (Fig. 3.26).

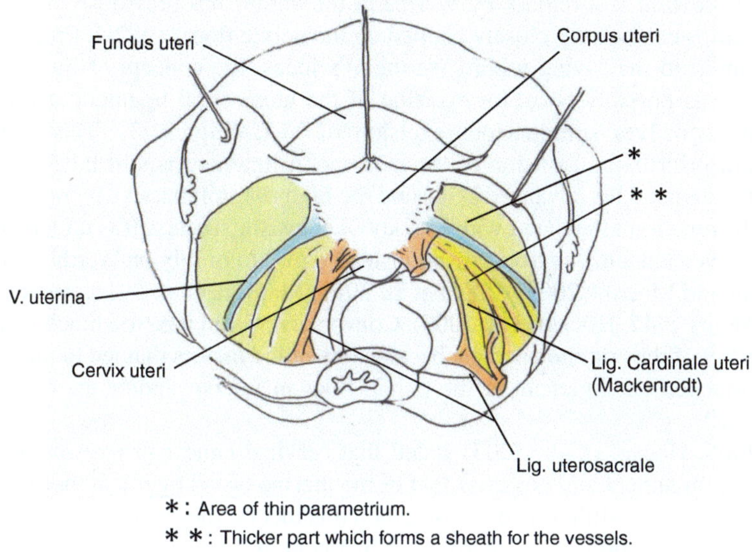

Fig. 3.26 Uterosacral ligament
This is a rough reproduction of Fig. 2.4 in the article by Curtis et al. (Surg Gyn Obst, 1940), with the ligamentous portions colored
Until around the mid-twentieth century, the uterosacral ligaments and TCL were considered to form a continuum, serving as an anchor connecting the uterine cervix and sacrum. Basis D, et al. named this complex "common pedicle." In 1950, Campbell classified the uterosacral ligament into three histological components: cervical, intermediate, and sacral, while Otcenasek in 2008 categorized it into vascular and neural parts and true uterosacral ligament. This concept can also be inferred from panel (**a**) of Fig. 2.23 in Wertheim's original article. However, in their classification, they did not introduce a concept for the lateral rectal ligament

Campbell (1950) also described the uterosacral ligament as consisting of cervical, intermediate, and sacral histological components. The 30th American edition of Gray's Anatomy (Clemente 1985) in 1985 stated: "The uterosacral ligament is a prominent fibrous band of subserous fascia that takes a curved course along the lateral wall of the pelvis from the cervix uteri to the sacrum. It is a posterior continuation of the tissue that forms the cardinal ligament."

Figure 3.26 is a drawing taken from an article published by Curtis et al. in 1940. Similarly, Campbell (1950) and Bastian and Lassau (1982) depicted the uterosacral ligament as a subserous figure observed from the medial, namely, the rectal, aspect of the ligament. Campbell et al. classified the uterosacral ligament based on histological observations into three types of tissue: cervical, or anterior third, intermediate, or middle third, and sacral, or posterior third. The author, however, believes that drawings by Curtis, Campbell, and Bastian were not observed from actual excavations of the pararectal space. Furthermore, they introduced no concept for the lateral rectal ligament. Therefore, the author speculates that the anterior third in Campbell's drawing may refer to TCL and the middle third to the lateral rectal ligament.

The following is a remark by Wertheim the author has previously quoted: "… these clamps can be very closely applied on the pelvic floor" (p. 26). From this, the author inferred that, lying within Wertheim's ideas, the concept of the "common pedicle" was possibly born, for excision of the uterosacral ligament at the pelvic floor also involves simultaneous excision of TCL (Fig. 2.23). This insight of Wertheim prioritizing excision of the uterosacral ligament is still inherited today. Given the demand for advanced skills and the high risks of massive hemorrhage and organ dysfunction associated with Latzko/Okabayashi surgery, it is understandable that there is a tendency to avoid it and instead return to or rely on Wertheim surgery (Querleu and Morrow 2008; Cibula et al. 2011; Magrina et al. 2011; Averette et al. 1993; Meigs 1945; Höckel et al. 2003). Conversely, would it be too much to ask that the concept of the common pedicle became one of the factors that led to the excision of the Mackenrodt ligament at the pelvic floor in Latzko and/or the Okabayashi procedure?

In 2005, Höckel et al. (2005) stated that cervical cancer progresses along the uterosacral ligament and posterior leaf of the uterine broad ligament, both of which originate from the Müllerian duct. Based on this theory, they proposed the necessity of extensive resection of the uterosacral ligament and posterior leaf of the uterine broad ligament in surgery for cervical cancer, which is defined as a total mesometrial resection (TMMR) (Höckel et al. 2003). Certainly, Kraima et al (2014). stated that one of the major pathways draining the uterine cervix is a dorsal pathway, running in the uterosacral ligament toward the rectal pillars.

The uterosacral ligament is unlikely to attach directly to the sacrum, or *periosteum*. Ercoli (Curtis et al. 1940) in 2005 mentioned that the uterosacral ligament merges with the parietal endopelvic fascia. Furthermore, Fritsch (Koster 1933) in 1992, a collaborator of Höckel, stated in a discussion of her article, "A structure which may be considered as a ligament, and which stretches from the uterus to the sacrum does not exist in fetuses. This finding is in agreement with the descriptions of Campell (1950) and Brizzi (1970) for the adult." Even if the uterosacral ligament attaches to the parietal endopelvic fascia, i.e., the superior fascia of the pelvic diaphragm, the lymphatic distribution of the endopelvic fascia is empirically very limited. In RH carried out by the author for FIGO stage IB2 cervical cancer, criteria for which was stipulated in 1998, recurrence at the resected stumps of the uterosacral ligaments and posterior leaf of the uterine broad ligament was found to be extremely rare with no evidence of metastasis to the parietal endopelvic fascia. According to the 3D MR scan analyses by Ramanah and/or DeLancy (Ramanah et al. 2012), in 73% of cases, the coccygeus muscle/sacrospinous ligament was found to be the origin for the uterosacral ligament.

In anatomic terms, the peritoneum of the Douglas pouch is referred to as the "rectouterine fold," whereas in Terminologia Anatomica, the terms "uterosacral ligament" and "rectouterine ligament" are considered synonymous. It can also be interpreted that the uterosacral ligament is the rectouterine ligament covered by the rectouterine fold (Fig. 4.23). Moreover, in Fig. 4.21, the rectouterine ligament is shown to form the inner aspect of the posterior mesoureter, fusing with the parietal endopelvic fascia at the lateral aspect of the sacrum. Does the uterosacral ligament exist in name only?

4 Clinical Anatomy of the Paracolpium

As mentioned in the section on the anterior support, the blood vessels of TCL and lateral rectal ligament reflect craniocaudally along the lateral aspect of each organ at their visceral termini (Figs. 3.15 and 3.24). The vessels descending caudally are accompanied by nerves, forming the paracolpium and paraproctium. Meanwhile, the blood vessels and nerves to the bladder, together with the anterior mesoureter, form the paracystium (Fig. 3.21).

Figure 3.27 depicts macroscopic and microscopic anatomic images of a coronal section of the superior-most vagina. Panel (**a**) shows a gross image sliced to a thickness of 2.5 cm. By the creation of the paravesical space and P&A's lower portion of the pararectal space, the superior fascia of the pelvic diaphragm lies between the two spaces. The tissue in panel (**b**) is stained with hematoxylin and eosin. In relation to the vagina, the anterior and posterior vaginal fasciae (red wedges on the right in Fig. 3.28) merge on the lateral edge to form the vaginal fascia, which covers the medial aspect of the neurovascular bundle, forming the paracolpium (within the black dashed lines in panels (**a**) and (**b**), as well as in Fig. 3.28).

Similarly, the paracystium (medial aspect of the red dashed lines) and paraproctium (medial aspect of the blue dashed lines) exhibit a similar morphology. Furthermore, the fascia of the lateral tissue of each organ converges at one point on the lateral aspect, as shown in Fig. 3.28, connecting to the tendinous arch of the pelvic fascia. It, then, connects with the superior fascia of the levator ani, ultimately reaching the tendinous arch of the levator ani. The superior fascia of the levator ani seen here corresponds to Mackenrodt's short fibrous bundle. Another significant observation is that, in panels (**a**) and (**b**) (also refer to panel (**b**) of Fig. 4.24), the paracystium, paracolpium, and paraproctium are demarcated by fascia, while in Fig. 3.8, which depicts SS, there are no clear boundaries between the three tissues composing SS. This suggests that the paracolpium and parametrium are morphologically and functionally distinct.

The black arrows in panel (**b**) of Fig. 3.27 indicate the path for creating the fourth space. The previously mentioned fourth space excavated between the uterine cervix and ureter (panel (**b**) of Figs. 3.13 and 3.19) demonstrates that simple extension and excavation is possible between the lateral margin of the vagina and anterior mesoureter (red arrow in panel (**a**) of Fig. 3.29 and yellow area in panel (**b**) of Fig. 3.29). A coronal section of the vagina shown in Fig. 3.28 illustrates the excavation of the fourth space along the red line, demonstrating the separation of the vesical nerve branches (Square b) and vaginal nerve branches (Square a).

There is a popular saying "the greater the amount of the vaginal excision, the worse the bladder paralysis." The creation of the fourth space has also resolved this issue. Furthermore, it can be inferred that the presence of the fourth space allows for an anatomic explanation for the formation of the birth canal. However, as the author is not an expert in this field, consulting the opinions of specialists is required.

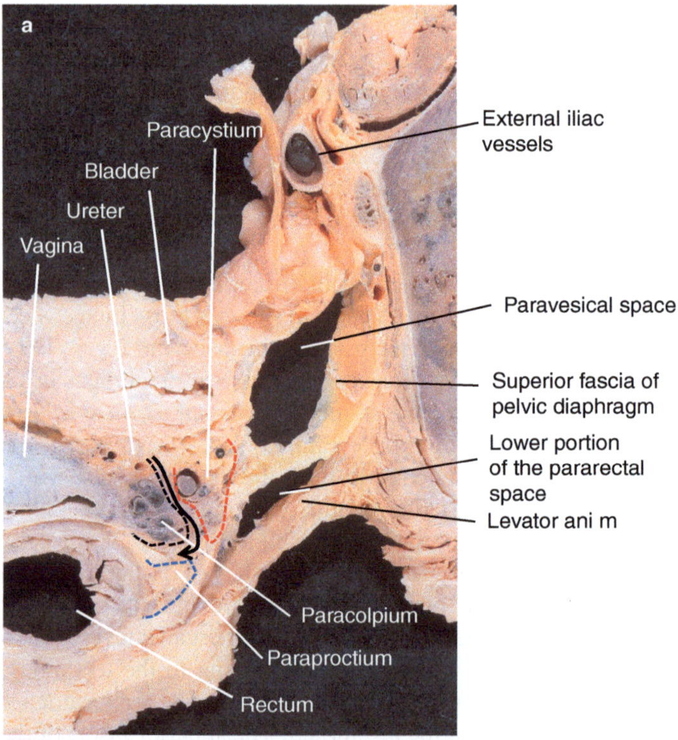
a
External iliac vessels
Paracystium
Bladder
Ureter
Vagina
Paravesical space
Superior fascia of pelvic diaphragm
Lower portion of the pararectal space
Levator ani m
Paracolpium
Paraproctium
Rectum

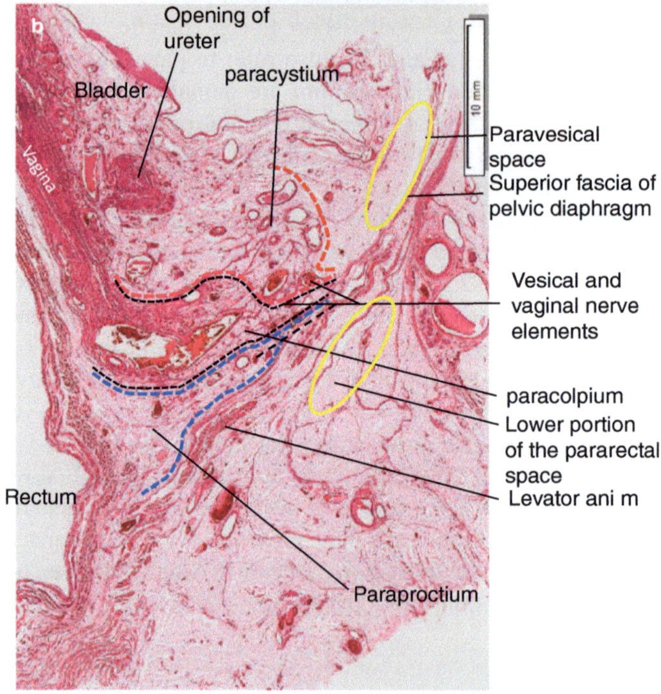
b
Opening of ureter
paracystium
Bladder
Vagina
10 mm
Paravesical space
Superior fascia of pelvic diaphragm
Vesical and vaginal nerve elements
paracolpium
Lower portion of the pararectal space
Levator ani m
Rectum
Paraproctium

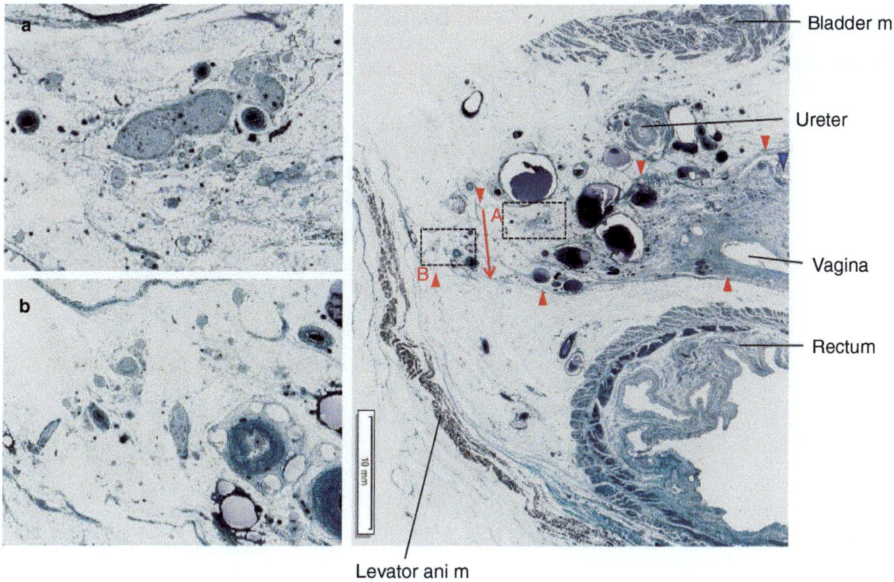

Fig. 3.28 Tissue image of the paracolpium
This tissue is stained with aldehyde-fuchsin. Square **a** corresponds to the region where the vaginal nerves are distributed, and Square **b** is considered to be the region of the pathway for the vesical nerve branch. The fourth space is excavated in a direction of the red arrow, separating the vesical nerve branch and vaginal nerve. The red wedges indicate the vaginal fascia

Fig. 3.27 Anatomy of the lateral vaginal ligament
Panel (**a**) is a coronally sectioned right half of the pelvis of a 76-year-old multipara donor, which is of 2.5-cm thickness showing the paracolpium and superior fascia of the pelvic diaphragm. The paravesical space and the lower portion of the pararectal space are seen created, and, between the spaces, the superior fascia of the pelvic diaphragm has been separated. The lateral edges, or fascia, of the paracystium (red dotted line), paracolpium (black dotted line), and paraproctium (blue dotted line) are seen to converge at the tendinous arch of the pelvic fascia, where they join the parietal endopelvic fascia, also known as the superior fascia of the pelvic diaphragm, terminating at the tendinous arc of the levator ani. The black curved arrow indicates the direction for the creation of the fourth space
Panel (**b**) shows a frontally sectioned histological tissue image with hematoxylin and eosin staining of the superior-most part of the vagina. The anterior and posterior vaginal fasciae are seen joined together at the lateral edge of the vagina to form the paracolpium. They, then, fuse with the fascia of the paracystium and paraproctium and connect to the superior fascia of the pelvic diaphragm. The area enclosed by the red line is the paracystium, the one by the black line the paracolpium, and that by the blue line the paraproctium. These regions are each independent and distinct, unlike the seamless continuity of the components in SS seen in Fig. 3.8. Please also refer to Fig. 4.38. (Reproduced from Yabuki 2023)

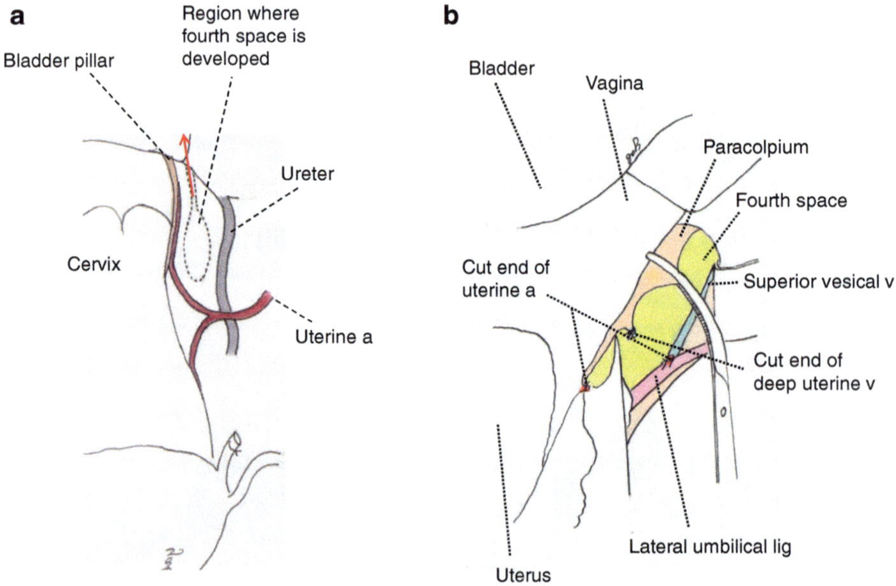

Fig. 3.29 Enlargement of the fourth space toward the perivagina
Schematic illustration in panel (**a**) shows that, by detaching the bladder, the fourth space can be extended caudally (red arrow)
Schematic illustration in panel (**b**) shows where the fourth space has been developed to the side of the vagina. The fourth space (area in yellow) is extended between the superior vesical vein and vagina with the paracolpium appearing on the medial aspect. This image depicts the paracolpium clamped with Kelly forceps in a direction to the right, as well as the fourth space, anterior mesoureter, paravesical space, and lateral umbilical ligament

5 Summary

The structure that connects the pelvic organs and pelvic sidewall consists of two bundles, one depicted by P&A horizontal to the organs shown in Fig. 2.1 and the other perpendicular depicted by the author in Fig. 3.6. Moreover, the latter is classified into three: SS, mesoureter, and suspensory system (Fig. 3.30).

SS represents a transversal vascular bundle that connects pelvic organs to the pelvic sidewall. It corresponds to a continuum consisting of the vesicohypogastric fascia, TCL, and lateral rectal ligament, which is an artifact that is severed following excavation of the paravesical and pararectal spaces. The suspensory system represents a longitudinal fascial ligament in which the pubocervical ligament, vesical fascia, vesicouterine ligament, cervical fascia, and uterosacral ligament connect from the pubis to the sacrum. Moreover, before intersecting the ureter, SS, including some of the blood vessels, reflects craniocaudally. The reflected portion forms a lamina, or neurovascular bundle, parallel to the pelvic autonomic nerve. The author terms this lamina as the mesoureter, which is dissected as an artifact that hangs from the ureter and located parallel with the suspensory system.

The horizontal bundle represents a horizontal continuum formed by the uterine broad ligament, CL, or Savage's "the condensation in the base of the broad

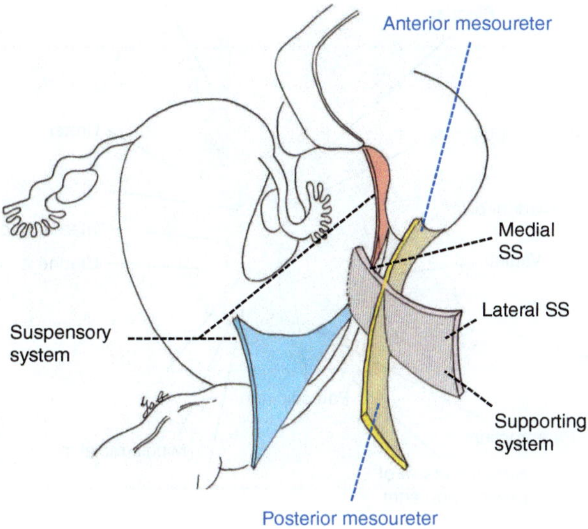

Fig. 3.30 Perpendicular bundle that appears in radical hysterectomy
This is a schematic summary of the bundle created perpendicularly to the subserous layer during surgery. This bundle consists of SS running mediolaterally, or transversally, and the mesoureter and suspensory system running craniocaudally, or *longitudinally*, intersecting at approximately a right angle. SS consists of the vesicohypogastric fascia, TCL, and lateral rectal ligament. The suspensory system and mesoureter do not form a complex. (Reproduced from Yabuki 2023)

ligament," and paracolpium (Figs. 3.27 and 3.31). As shown in Figs. 3.5, 3.12, and 3.27, the paracolpium combines with the superior fascia of the pelvic diaphragm, together with the paracystium, and paraproctium to connect a part of the pelvic floor. As shown in Figs. 2.12 and 2.27, CL, which is connective tissue connecting the ureter and the lateral edge of the uterine cervix, connects to the uterine broad ligament via the uterine ascending vessel branch, forming the horizontal continuum via the descending vessel branch. TCL corresponds to a part of the perpendicular continuum, or *SS*, formed in parallel with the superior vesical artery, uterine vessels, and middle rectal vessels (Fig. 3.9). CL and TCL intersect on the medial aspect of the ureter, forming "the condensation" (Fig. 3.31), which causes difficulty in excising TCL during RH (Fig. 3.15). To resolve this problem, four spaces are excavated around the intersection of TCL and mesoureter shown in Fig. 3.32.

In Fig. 2.1 by P&A, the transitional zone is depicted as a blank, and the author has proposed as shown in Fig. 3.8, that it is possible to fit SS into it. Figure 3.31 depicts the horizontal bundle and SS, the latter of which is the perpendicular bundle. The author concludes that the lateral ligaments of the pelvic organs are a combination of structures shown in Figs. 3.30 and 3.31. It can be inferred from each of the organs' description by P&A that the frontal connective tissue ground bundle corresponds to the intraperitoneal structure, and the horizontal connective tissue ground bundle corresponds to the extraperitoneal structure. The boundary between the two ground bundles is termed the intermediary part that corresponds to the ventrodorsal vascular bundle, or SS advocated by the author (Fig. 3.8). Looking from this

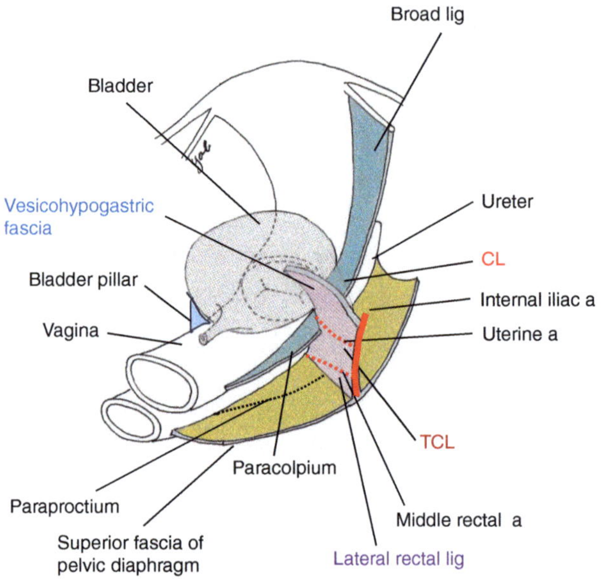

Fig. 3.31 Horizontal bundle that appears in radical hysterectomy
The horizontal bundle that appears during surgery corresponds to a continuum consisting of the uterine broad ligament, CL, or the condensation in the base of the uterine broad ligament of Savage, and paracolpium. As shown in Figs. 3.5, 3.12, and 3.27, the paracolpium combines with the superior fascia of the pelvic diaphragm together with the paracystium and paraproctium, forming the pelvic floor. This figure depicts findings of this horizontal bundle intersecting with the perpendicular SS at the uterine cervix. The ureter/mesoureter exist on the lateral aspect where both bundles intersect (Fig. 3.30). Therefore, one can see the clinical anatomy of this surrounding area is very complex. (Reproduced from Yabuki 2023)

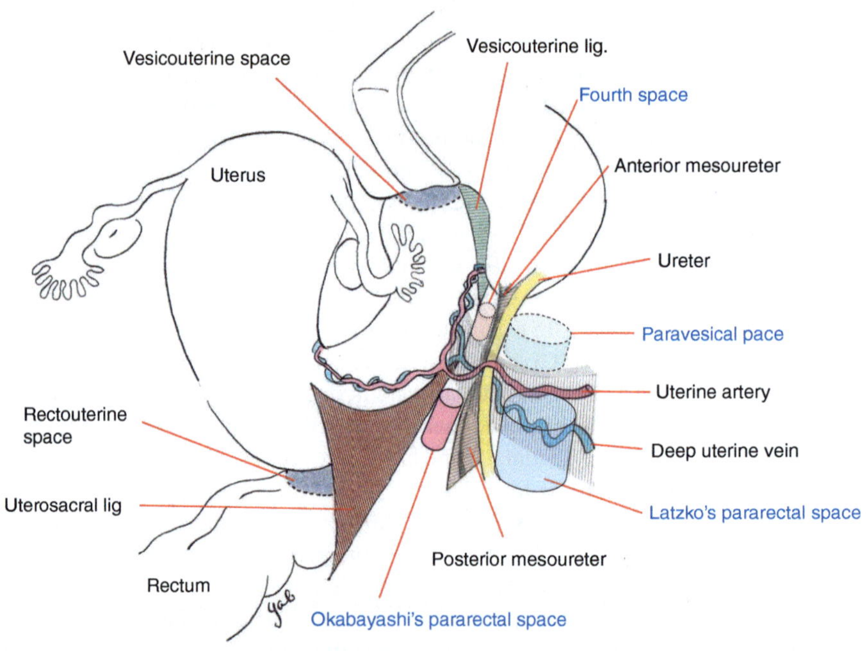

Fig. 3.32 Artificial spaces appearing during surgical procedures
This diagram emphasizes the spaces excavated in the subserous layer during RH. These spaces are excavated along the bundles in a direction of the sacrum. (Reproduced from Yabuki 2023)

perspective, it would be feasible to integrate P&A's theory, or basic anatomy, with clinical anatomy acquired by the author during surgery.

In this chapter, the author has attempted to introduce a three-dimensional clinical anatomy to classical anatomy expressed and interpreted within a two-dimensional basic anatomy. From this, a successful outcome has been achieved regarding post-operative preservation of bladder function and a decrease in intraoperative hemorrhaging, issues that have long lingered since the time of L&S.

References

Averette HE, Nguyen HN, Donato DM et al (1993) Radical hysterectomy for invasive cervical cancer: a 25-year prospective experience with the Miami technique. Cancer Suppl 71:1422–1437. PMID: 8431876. https://doi.org/10.1002/cncr.2820710407

Bastian D, Lassau JP (1982) The suspensory mechanism of the uterus: anatomical basis for the statics and dynamics of the normal uterus. Anat Clin 4:147–160

Berglas B, Rubin IC (1953) Histologic study of the pelvic connective tissue. Surg Gynecol Obstet 97(277–87):449. PMID: 13090052

Blaisdell FE (1917) The anatomy of the sacrouterine ligaments. Anat Rec 12:1–42

Campbell RM (1950) Anatomy and histology of the sacrouterine ligament. Am J Obstet Gynecol 59:1–12. PMID: 15399622. https://doi.org/10.1016/0002-9378(50)90334-6

Cibula D, Abu-Rustum NR, Benedetti-Panici P et al (2011) New classification system of radical hysterectomy: emphasis on a three-dimensional anatomic template for parametrial resection. Gynecol Oncol 122:264–268. PMID: 21592548. Epub 2011 May 17. https://doi.org/10.1016/j.ygyno.2011.04.029

Clemente CD (ed) (1985) Anatomy of the human body by Henry Gray, 30th American ed, vol 1. Lea & Febiger, Philadelphia, pp 1574–1577

Curtis AH, Anson BJ, Beaton LE (1940) The anatomy of the subperitoneal tissues and ligamentous structures in relation to surgery of the female pelvic viscera. Surg Gyn Obstet 70:643–656

Drake RL, Vogl W, Mitchell AWM (eds) (2005) Gray's anatomy for students. Elsevier, Philadelphia

Ercoli A, Delmas V, Fanfani F et al (2005) Terminology Anatomica versus unofficial descriptions and nomenclature of the fasciae and ligaments of the female pelvis: a dissection-based comparative study. Am J Obstet Gynecol 193:1565–1573. PMID: 16202758. https://doi.org/10.1016/j.ajog.2005.05.007

Fritsch H (1992) The connective tissue sheath of uterus and vagina in the human female fetus. Ann Anat 174:261–266. PMID: 150324. https://doi.org/10.1016/s0940-9602(11)80366-3

Goff BH (1931) Histological study of perivaginal fascia in a nullipara. Surg Gynecol Obstet 443(52):32–42

Greenhill JP, Friedman. (1974) Biological principles and modern practice of obstetrics. WB Saunders Co, Philadelphia, p 110

Höckel M, Horn LC, Hentschel B et al (2003) Total mesometrial resection: high resolution nerve-sparing radical hysterectomy based on developmentally defined surgical anatomy. Int J Gynecol Cancer 13:791–803. PMID: 14675316. https://doi.org/10.1111/j.1525-1438.2003.13608.x

Höckel M, Horn LC, Fritsch H (2005) Association between the mesenchymal compartment of uterovaginal organogenesis and local tumor spread in stage IB-IIB cervical carcinoma: a prospective study. Lancet Oncol 6:751–756. PMID: 16198980. https://doi.org/10.1016/S1470-2045(05)70324-7

Howkins J, Stallworthy J (1974) Bonny's gynaecological surgery, 8th edn. Bailliere Tindall, London

Kocks J (1880) Die Normale und Pathologische Lage und Gestalt des Uterus Sowie deren Mechanik. Max Cohen & Sohn, Bonn

Koster H (1933) On the supports of the uterus. Am J Obstet Gynecol 25:67–74

Kraima AC, Derks M, Smit NN et al (2014) Lymphatic drainage pathways from the cervix uteri: implications for radical hysterectomy? Gynecol Oncol 132(1):107–113. PMID: 24201016. https://doi.org/10.1016/j.ygyno.2013.10.030

Mackenrodt A (1895) Ueber die Ursachen der normalen und pathologischen Lagen des Uterus. Arch F Gynäk 48:393–421

Magrina JF, Pawlina W, Kho RM et al (2011) Robotic nerve-sparing radical hysterectomy: feasibility and technique. Gynecol Oncol 121:605–609. PMID: 21419478. https://doi.org/10.1016/j.ygyno.2011.02.034

Meigs JV (1945) Wertheim operation for carcinoma of cervix. Am J Obstet Gynecol 49:542–553

Niikura H, Katahira A, Utsunomiya H et al (2007) Surgical anatomy of intrapelvic fascia and vesico-uterine ligament in nerve-sparing radical hysterectomy with fresh cadaver dissections. Tohoku J Exp Med 212:403–413. PMID: 17660706. https://doi.org/10.1620/tjem.212.403

Peham HV, Amreich J (1930) Gynäkologische Operationslehre. VERLAG VON S. KARGER, BASEL

Peham HV, Amreich J (1934) Operative gynecology, vol. 2 (translated by Ferguson LK). JB Lippincott, Philadelphia, pp 333–366

Pick TP, Howden R (eds) (1901) Gray's anatomy: descriptive and surgical, 15th edn. Barnes & Noble, New York, pp 1012–1014

Querleu D, Morrow CP (2008) Classification of radical hysterectomy. Lancet Oncol 9:297–303. PMID:18308255. https://doi.org/10.1016/S1470-2045(08)70074-3

Ramanah R, Berger MB, Parratte BM et al (2012) Anatomy and histology of apical support: a literature review concerning cardinal and uterosacral ligament. Int Urogynecol J 23:1483–1494. PMID: 22618209 PMCID: PMC4258694. https://doi.org/10.1007/s00192-012-1819-7

Range RL, Woodburne RT (1964) The gross and microscopic anatomy of the transverse cervical ligament. Am J Obstet Gynecol 90:460–467. PMID: 14217646. https://doi.org/10.1016/0002-9378(64)90802-6

Raspagliesi F, Ditto A, Fontanelli R et al (2004) Nerve-sparing radical hysterectomy: a surgical technique for preserving the autonomic hypogastric nerve. Gynecol Oncol 93:307–314. PMID: 15099938. https://doi.org/10.1016/j.ygyno.2004.01.048

Reiffenstuhl G (1964) The lymphatics of the female organs. JB Lippincott, Philadelphia

Reiffenstuhl G (1982) The clinical significance of the connective tissue planes and spaces. Clin Obstet Gynecol 25:812–820

Rock JA, Thompson JA (1996) Te Linde's operative gynecology, 8th edn. Lippincott-Raven, Philadelphia/New York

Sato K, Sato T (1991) The vascular and neuronal composition of the lateral ligament of the rectum and the rectosacral fascia. Surg Radiol Anat 13:17–22. PMID: 2053040. https://doi.org/10.1007/BF01623135

Savage H (1870) The surgery, surgical pathology, and surgical anatomy of the female pelvic organ, 3rd edn. J & A Churchill & Son, London, p 76

Uhlenhuth E, Day DE, Smith RD et al (1948) The visceral endopelvic fascia and the hypogastric sheath. Surg Gynecol Obstet 86:9–28. PMID: 18920874

Yabuki Y (2016) Clinical anatomy of the subserous layer: an amalgamation of gross and clinical anatomy. Clin Anat 29:508–515

Yabuki Y (2020) Twenty-first century radical hysterectomy: journey from descriptive to practical anatomy. Gynecol Oncol Rep 34:100623

Yabuki Y (2023) Two lateral parametria in radical hysterectomy: history and outcome. J Obstet Gynecol Res. 43:1069–1078

Yabuki Y, Asamoto A, Hoshiba T et al (1991) Dissection of the cardinal ligament in radical hysterectomy for cervical cancer with emphasis on the lateral ligament. Am J Obstet Gynecol 164:7–14. PMID: 1986630. https://doi.org/10.1016/0002-9378(91)90614-w

Yabuki Y, Asamoto A, Hoshiba T et al (1996) A new proposal for radical hysterectomy. Gynecol Oncol 62:370–378. PMID: 8812535. [PubMed]. https://doi.org/10.1006/gyno.1996.0251

Yabuki Y et al (2005) Discrepancies between classic anatomy and modern gynecologic surgery on pelvic connective tissue structure: harmonization of those concepts by collaborative cadaver dissection. Am J Obstet Gynecol 193:7–15

Yabuki Y et al (2011) Redefinition of the pelvic connective tissue: in-situ histologic examination. Female Pelvic Med & Reconstr Surg 17:60–66

Chapter 4
Surgical Procedures

Abbreviations

CL	Cardinal ligament
IFFA	International Federation of Associations of Anatomists
IHP	Inferior hypogastric plexus
L&S	Latzko and Schiffmann
LP	Lateral parametrium
LUL	Lateral umbilical ligament
NSRH	Nerve-sparing radical hysterectomy
P&A	Peham-Americh
PSN	Pelvic splanchnic nerve
Q&M	Querleu and Morrow
RH	Radical hysterectomy
TA	Terminologia Anatomica
TCL	Transverse cervical ligament
TMMR	Total mesometrial resection
VUL	Vesicouterine ligament

Characteristics of the author's RH procedure involve preservation of the bladder and rectal function with non-excision of the lateral rectal ligament. For this, the following is carried out: (a) perpendicular excavation of the paravesical space, Latzko's pararectal space, fourth space, and Okabayashi's pararectal space and (b) excision of (i) SS, or *a complex consisting of the vesicohypogastric fascia, TCL, and lateral rectal ligament*, (ii) the mesoureter that is *separated into anterior and posterior parts*, and (iii) the suspensory system consisting of *the uterosacral and vesicouterine ligaments*, all of which are selectively separated by the creation of the perpendicularly created spaces. All photographs in this chapter were taken during surgery unless otherwise stated.

The original version of the chapter has been revised. A correction to this chapter can be found at https://doi.org/10.1007/978-981-96-7194-6_5

Y. Yabuki, *Nerve-Sparing Radical Hysterectomy*,
https://doi.org/10.1007/978-981-96-7194-6_4

1 Sequence of the Surgical Procedure for Nerve-Sparing Radical Hysterectomy

1.1 Abdominal Incision

1.2 Division of the Round Ligament of the Uterus

The round ligament should be severed as distally as possible with incision of the parietal peritoneum extending from the lateral edge of the divided round ligament to the bifurcation of the common iliac vessels (Fig. 4.1). At this time, excision of the infundibulopelvic ligament is not carried out.

1.3 Excavation of the Retroperitoneal Space

Pulling on the lateral suture of the uterine round ligament, insert the tips of both index fingers between the parietal peritoneum and psoas major muscle, and then spread the fingers apart to separate the peritoneum, exposing the external iliac artery up to the common iliac artery (panel (**a**) of Fig. 4.2).

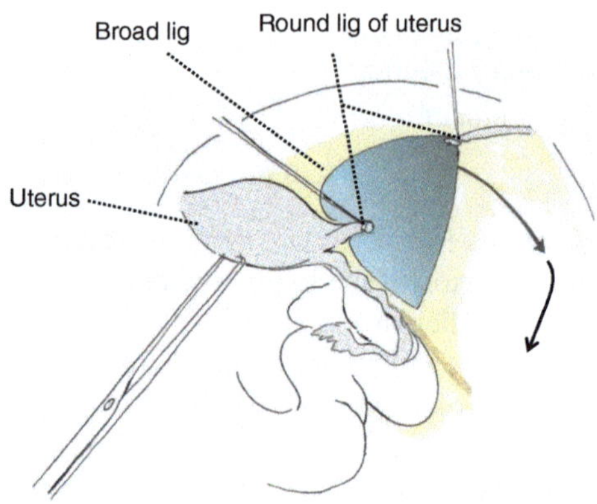

Fig. 4.1 Schematic illustration to demonstrate severance of the round ligament and incision of the iliac fossa peritoneum
Separate the round ligament on its lateral aspect, pull up the thread of the lateral ligature, insert the fingers into the incision so as to separate the peritoneum from the iliopsoas muscle, and then extend the peritoneal incision cranially along the psoas major muscle (arrows), which results in the appearance of the triangular preovarian fossa, also known as Waldeyer's fossa. (Reproduced from Yabuki 2019, 2023)

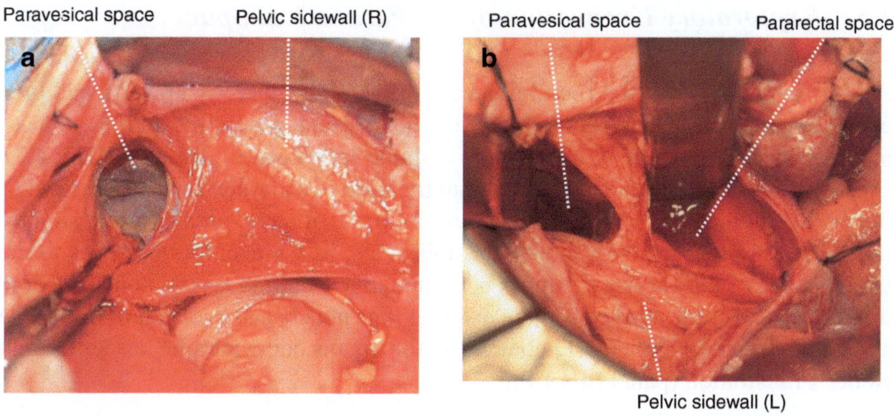

Fig. 4.2 Exposure of the psoas major muscle and exploratory excavation of the paravesical and pararectal spaces
Shown are the right and left pelvic cavities from the mediocranial aspects. The psoas major muscle is seen detached from the parietal peritoneum with an exploratory excavation of the pararectal and paravesical spaces having taken place, revealing the separated TCL on the left pelvic sidewall

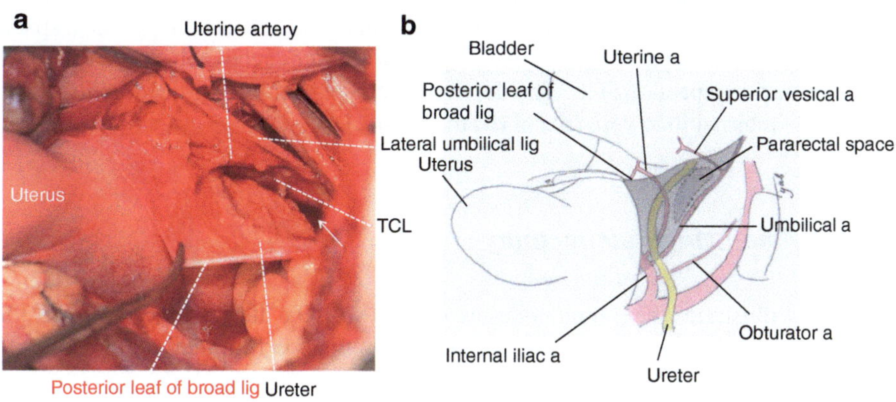

Fig. 4.3 Development of the uterine broad ligament and exposure of the ureter
Panel (**a**) shows an intraoperative photograph of the development of Latzko's pararectal space (arrow). The posterior leaf of the uterine broad ligament and lateral umbilical ligament are seen being pulled with forceps, respectively. Following this, visual confirmation is required for the course of the ureter attached to the posterior leaf of the uterine broad ligament up to the entrance of ureteric tunnel
Panel (**b**) is a schematic explanation

1.4 Exposure of the Ureter

The ureter enters the pelvic cavity caudal to the bifurcation of the common iliac artery into the internal and external iliac arteries, and its course can be observed by lifting the posterior leaf of the uterine broad ligament while attached to this ligament, passing behind TCL (Fig. 4.3).

1.5 Exploratory Excavation of the Paravesical Space

Pull the outer suture of the round ligament of the uterus directly upward, and then using the fingertips or scissors to locate the nonresistant part of the areolar connective tissue directly beneath, use a sharp or blunt technique to dissect it (Fig. 4.2). This excavation can be carried out without the need to excavate down to the level of the levator ani muscle. While excavating with the fingers, areas with a slightly fibrous texture may be encountered. At this stage, as the excavation moves to the lateral space of the vagina, it should be terminated. Through lymph node excision, the paravesical space connects to the external iliac pouch, and excision of this space should proceed perpendicularly contrary to the organs being parallel, as depicted in Netter's illustration (panel (**a**) of Fig. 2.3).

1.6 Exploratory Excavation of Latzko's Pararectal Space

To visualize the course of the ureter (Fig. 4.3), the incised edge of the posterior leaf of the uterine broad ligament is lifted with forceps and commencing from the entrance to the ureteric tunnel in a laterocranial direction, proceed to create a space by gently pushing, separating, and excising the areolar connective tissue that adheres to the posterior aspect of TCL. The depth of excision should be guided by the location of the internal iliac vein (panel (**b**) of Fig. 4.2).

1.7 Pelvic Lymphadenectomy

Figure 4.4 illustrates the lymph nodes associated with the uterine cervix. Figure 3.9 shows the distribution of blood vessels within the pelvis following completion of pelvic lymphadenectomy.

Reiffenstuhl's classification (Reiffenstuhl 1964) of the pelvic lymph nodes was adopted until the 1900s, and the ones he identified as having the highest frequency of metastasis in cervical cancer were the interiliac lymph nodes and superior and inferior gluteal lymph nodes. Reiffenstuhl also stated that the lymphatic vessels extending from the base of the parametrium to the pelvic wall drain into the inferior gluteal lymph nodes. However, Reiffenstuhl's base of the parametrium refers to the base of the lateral rectal ligament. Therefore, this theory can be considered as being applicable to the pathway for lymphatic metastasis in rectal cancer (Fig. 2.16). This lack of clear distinction between TCL and the lateral rectal ligament is a good example of how confusion can arise.

Table 4.1 shows the distribution of sentinel lymph nodes, cited from a review by Cibula D and Abu-Rustum (Gynecol Oncol, 2010).

The author carries out lymph node dissection in the following order, but it is changeable depending on circumstances.

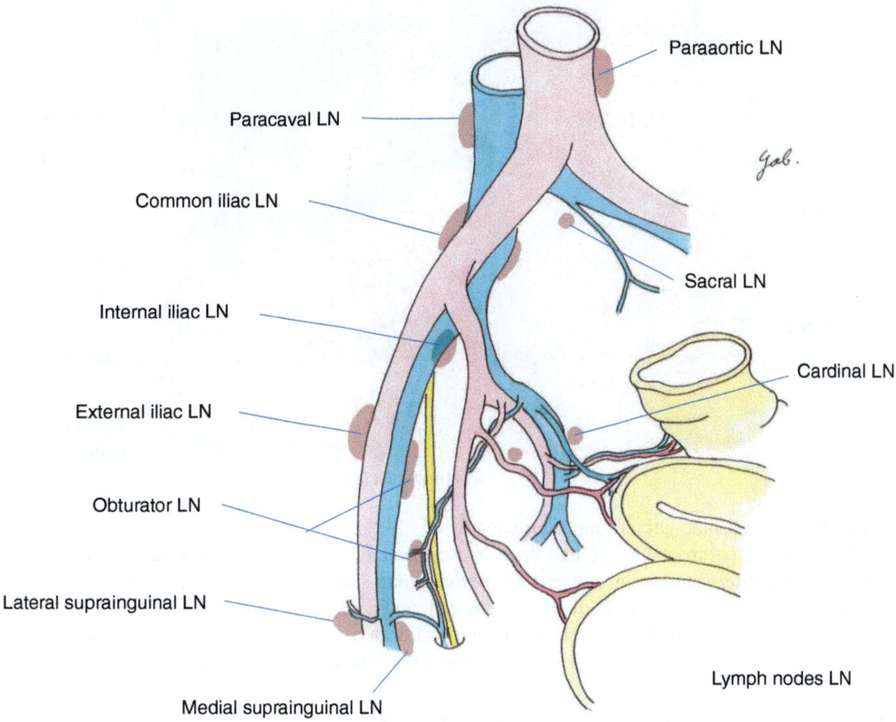

Fig. 4.4 Lymph nodes of the uterine cervix
This schematic illustration indicates the lymph nodes that may be excised during surgery for cervical cancer

Table 4.1 Metastatic distribution of sentinel nodes by Cibula (2010)

Region	Distribution of SN in %	Positive SN in %	Positive LN in %
Common iliac	5	5–7	7-36
Presacral	5	5	–
External iliac	5–47	39–46	4–45
Obturator	35–70	41–46	18–86
Internal iliac	3–8	0	9–15

1.7.1 Separation of the External Iliac Vessels from the Psoas Major Muscle

Proceed with the separation of the external iliac vessels and psoas major muscle at a uniform depth along their entire length (Fig. 4.5). Pull the vessels medially and continue separating the loose connective tissue until the obturator nerve becomes visible. As one approaches the inguinal region, the connective tissue may become slightly denser, but overall, the excision should remain relatively easy. This area is referred to as the obturator fossa.

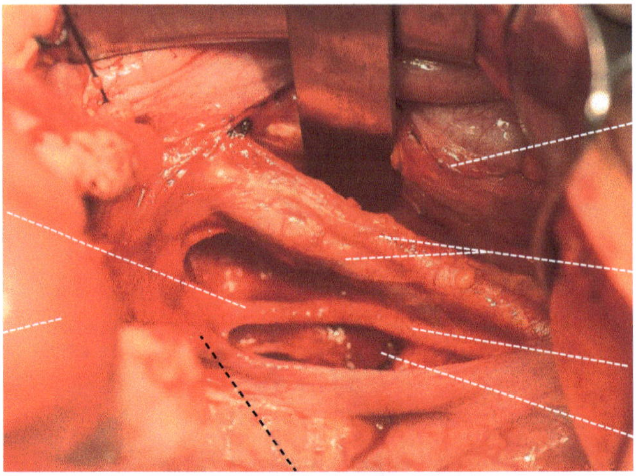

Fig. 4.5 External iliac vessels and their sheath
In this case, the pararectal space had been test-excavated, revealing the internal iliac artery. The external iliac artery and vein covered by perivascular sheaths are seen exposed with the area between the psoas major muscle already separated, and a retractor seen inserted. When the vascular sheath of the internal iliac vessels and posterior fascia of TCL are, respectively, separated from their main bodies, the pararectal space, or Latzko's pararectal space, naturally unfolds

1.7.2 Clearance of the External Iliac Vessels

Lymph node excision basically involves denuding the perivascular sheath from around the blood vessels in an en bloc resection.

As shown in Figs. 4.6 and 4.7, the author's technique involves progressing the dissection caudally by incising along the long axis of the vessels and separating the perivascular sheath from the entire circumference of the vessels. First, make a small incision in the perivascular sheath approximately 2–3 cm cranially to the bifurcation of the common iliac artery, then extend the incision caudally, gradually separating it (panel (**b**) of Fig. 4.6). At this time, if the deep iliac circumflex vein draining into the external iliac vein is identified as climbing over the external iliac artery, and therefore exposed, the procedure is temporarily halted (Fig. 4.8).

Next, as shown in panel (**a**) of Fig. 4.6, an incision is made into the perivascular sheath of the external iliac vein, and a similar procedure is carried out. However, caution is required when separating the sheath of the detached vein from the underlying tissue (panel (**c**)). In particular, numerous tributaries from the psoas major muscle or the superior gluteal vein converge on the posterior aspect of the bifurcation of the common iliac vein. The iliolumbar branch to/from the psoas major muscle is frequently encountered at two locations. One location is slightly caudal to where the external iliac vessels are buried in fat, and the other approximately 2–3 cm cranially to the inguinal region, although Gray's Anatomy for Students (Drake et al. 2005) states that there are no corresponding veins to the iliolumbar artery branching from the posterior trunks of the internal iliac vessels. However, this area still requires careful attention. While there are no veins running alongside the umbilical artery,

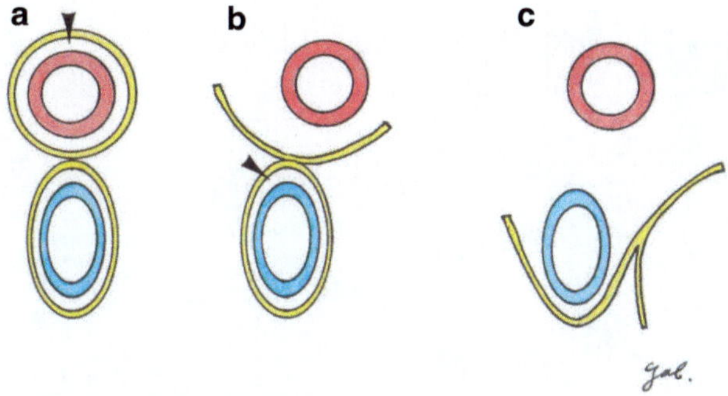

Fig. 4.6 The method for lymph node excision
This illustration shows the method for separation of the vascular sheath from the external iliac artery/vein
Panel (**a**): An incision (arrowhead) is made in the arterial vascular sheath
Panel (**b**): Separate the artery from the entire circumference of the sheath. Then, make an incision (arrowhead) into the venous vascular sheath
Panel (**c**): Separate the venous vascular sheath from the entire circumference of the vein while leaving the arterial vascular sheath attached

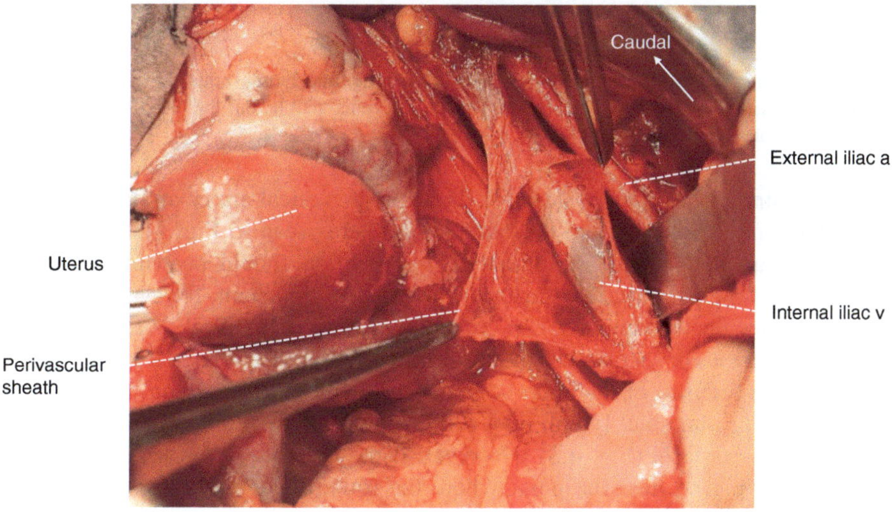

Fig. 4.7 Exposure of the external iliac vein
Here, one side of the incised vascular sheath is held by the assistant, and using Kelly forceps, it is incised and separated in a craniocaudal direction. When removing it from strongly adhered areas on the vein, utilize an opening and closing force of dressing forceps. If its damage to the nutrient vessels occurs, it may result in the formation of a hematoma beneath the fascia, but serious consequences from this are rare. However, greater caution is required for removal on the posterior aspect of the vein and at the transitional point of the femoral ring

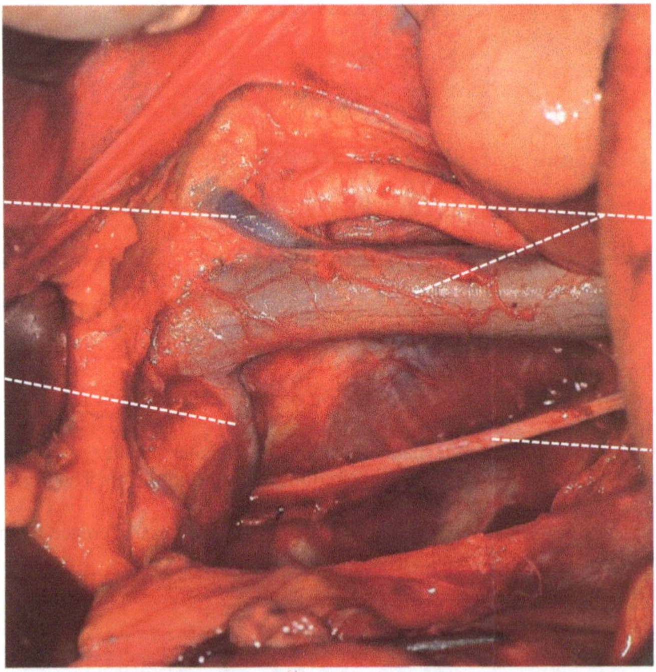

Fig. 4.8 Excision of the medial suprainguinal lymph nodes
This photograph shows that the clearance of the suprainguinal lymph nodes is nearly complete with the accessory obturator and deep iliac circumflex veins visible, but the lateral suprainguinal lymph nodes are still not cleared

there is a similar drainage system for the superior vesical artery as shown in Fig. 3.21. This may correspond to the unidentified veins seen in Figs. 4.10 and 4.11, possibly equivalent to the iliolumbar vein. Attention should be paid during the separation of the perivascular sheath of the external iliac vein, for even extremely fine blood vessels, if damaged, can create a hematoma (Fig. 4.7). While this does not lead to serious consequences, it can contribute to intraoperative anxiety.

Following removal of the node-bearing fatty tissue of the external iliac vessels, the lateral supra-inguinal lymph nodes are frequently not removed due to the low incident of metastasis (Fig. 4.8). However, if they are required to be removed, a hook can be placed near the point where the round ligament enters the inguinal region, and strong traction applied in a laterocaudal direction to expose them as they are enveloped in abundant fat. This fatty mass is then grasped with forceps, pulled anteriorly, and carefully excised with scissors from the surrounding pelvic wall tissues. During excision, meticulous ligation is carried out to prevent postoperative pelvic lymphocyst.

1.7.3 Excision of the Medial Supra-inguinal Lymph Nodes

The external iliac artery is lifted, and the medial supra-inguinal lymph nodes with the fatty tissue are grasped with forceps and pulled forward and ligated and severed in the inguinal region (Fig. 4.8). The excised medial supra-inguinal lymph nodes are passed under the accessory obturator vein that exits the obturator foramen and drains into the external iliac vein (no need to insist on passing these nodes underneath) and then gathered with the previously cleared external iliac nodes (Fig. 4.8).

1.7.4 Excision of the Obturator Lymph Nodes

The obturator fossa is an area filled with abundant fatty-areolar connective tissue, including a slightly concave region containing small lymph nodes, centered around the course of the obturator nerve (Fig. 4.9). The lateral aspect of the obturator fossa is formed by the fascia of the obturator internus muscle, while the medial aspect is the paravesical space/vesicohypogastric fascia. It extends caudally to the obturator foramen, and cranially to the origin of the lateral ligament or bifurcation of the common iliac vessels, or the triangles of iliac vessels (Figs. 4.9, 4.10, 4.13, 4.14, and 4.15).

This dissection involves using an intestinal retractor or hook to widely expand the area between the external iliac vessels and psoas major muscle (Fig. 4.9). First, the obturator nerve is identified exiting the obturator foramen and then separated

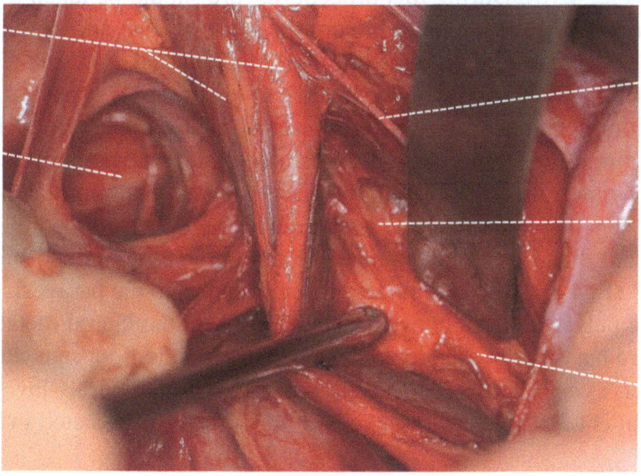

Fig. 4.9 The development and clearance of the obturator fossa
The external iliac vessels that have been separated from the psoas major muscle are pulled either toward the operator's side or medially, and the muscle is further pressed and displaced by the use of a 2–3-cm wide malleable retractor, thereby progressing deeper to separate these vessels and the muscle. In the photograph, the obturator nerve remains buried within the fat. With a small sponge held in a forceps, the nerve can be exposed through the obturator foramen in a manner similar to that used for removal of the fat. When the nerve cannot be found, excavation has often tended to come too close to the pelvic wall. Here, the paravesical space appears to be significantly developed medially

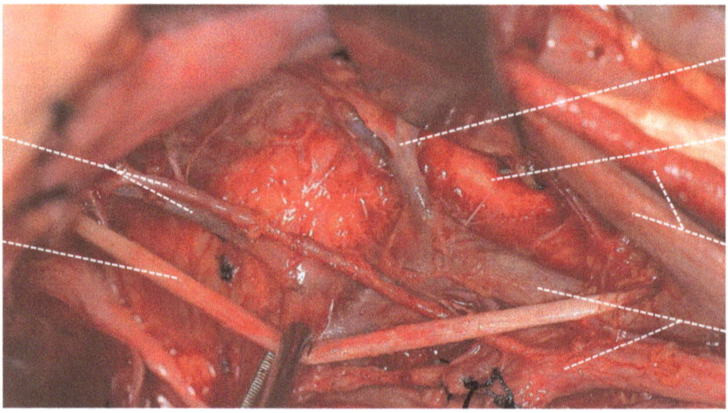

Fig. 4.10 View of the cleared obturator fossa
In the center of the photograph, the obturator nerve and accompanying artery and vein are seen to run in parallel. The obturator and deep uterine veins are seen to converge in close proximity to one another and drain into the internal iliac vein. In the iliac triangle, the lumbosacral trunk that becomes a landmark for the depth of clearance can be seen between the internal and external iliac veins. The umbilical artery can be seen excised at its base

from its surrounding tissues and is to be used as a landmark (Fig. 4.10). Next, while protecting the nerve and by the use of a technique incorporating liposuction dissection, the obturator vessels, which run along the laterodorsal aspect of the nerve, are separated from the fatty-areolar connective tissue until they drain into the internal iliac vessels (Fig. 4.10). During this procedure, care should be taken to avoid damaging the parietal perforating branch from the internal iliac and obturator vessels. The deep uterine and obturator veins drain into the internal iliac vein (Fig. 4.11).

This area of manipulation, which connects to the posterior aspect of the bifurcation of the common iliac vein, requires utmost caution. Therefore, it is recommended to approach this region not only from one direction but alternative directions such as the common iliac vein. The fatty tissue mass containing the excised small lymph nodes is gathered together with the previously collected medial supra-inguinal and external iliac lymph nodes near the obturator foramen and brought to the origin of TCL (Fig. 4.12). The obturator fossa connects to the paravesical space and extends to the pelvic floor. In conventional RH, where the lateral rectal ligament is removed, there have been cases reported where the pelvic floor muscles and pelvic splanchnic nerves are exposed. However, in procedures that purely involve the excision of TCL, it is advisable to limit excision to the level as depicted in Fig. 4.11.

1.7.5 Excision of the Internal Iliac Lymph Nodes

The internal iliac lymph nodes are located at the bifurcation of the external and internal iliac vessels, known as the triangle of iliac vessels. This area overlaps with the region of the origin of TCL (Figs. 4.10, 4.13, 4.14 and 4.15). When clearing this vascular triangle, it is extremely difficult to completely detach the posterior, or *dorsal*, surface of the venous triangle from the pelvic wall, as it is fixated by the posterior

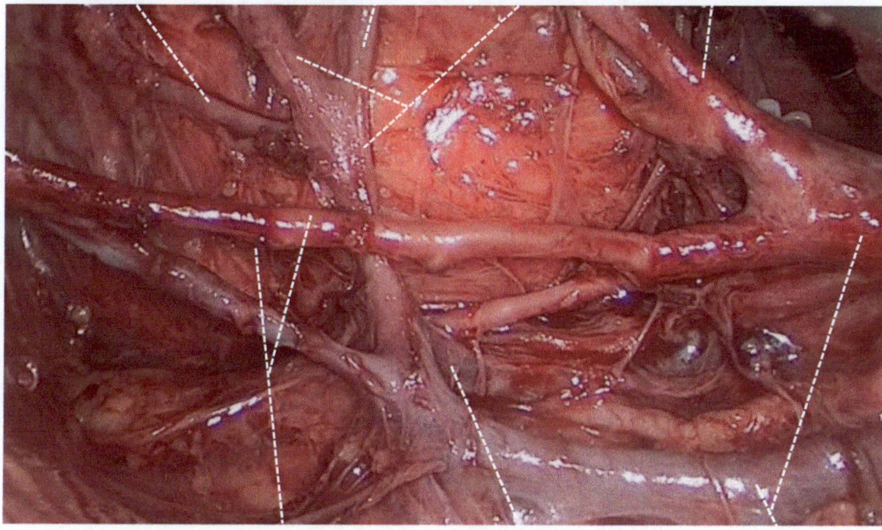

Fig. 4.11 Lateral dissection of the pelvis
This dissection shows procedure carried out by laparoscopic surgery. The iliac fossa is seen exposed, and the vessels at the origin of TCL are separated. The obturator and deep uterine veins converge into the internal iliac vein with venous blood from the bladder, uterus, and vagina draining into the deep uterine vein. (By courtesy of Tsutomu Hoshiba, MD, PhD., my most capable and trustworthy colleague)

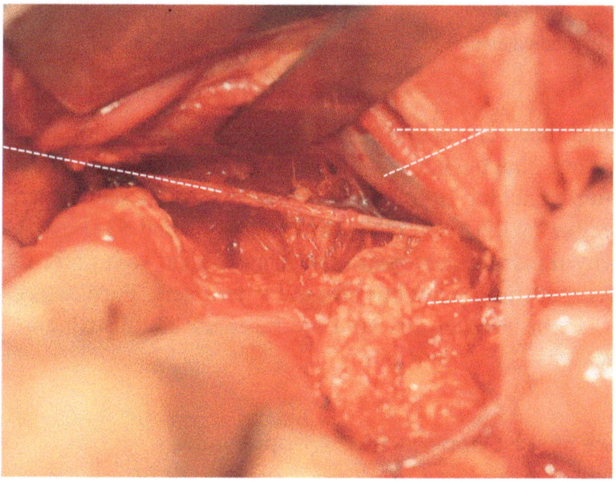

Fig. 4.12 Collection of node-bearing fatty tissue
This shows an en bloc excision of the external iliac nodes, internal and external suprainguinal nodes, and obturator nodes, which are seen gathered at the base of the lateral umbilical ligament. The obturator artery/vein, as well as the vessels penetrating their parietal aspect, is hidden behind the obturator nerve

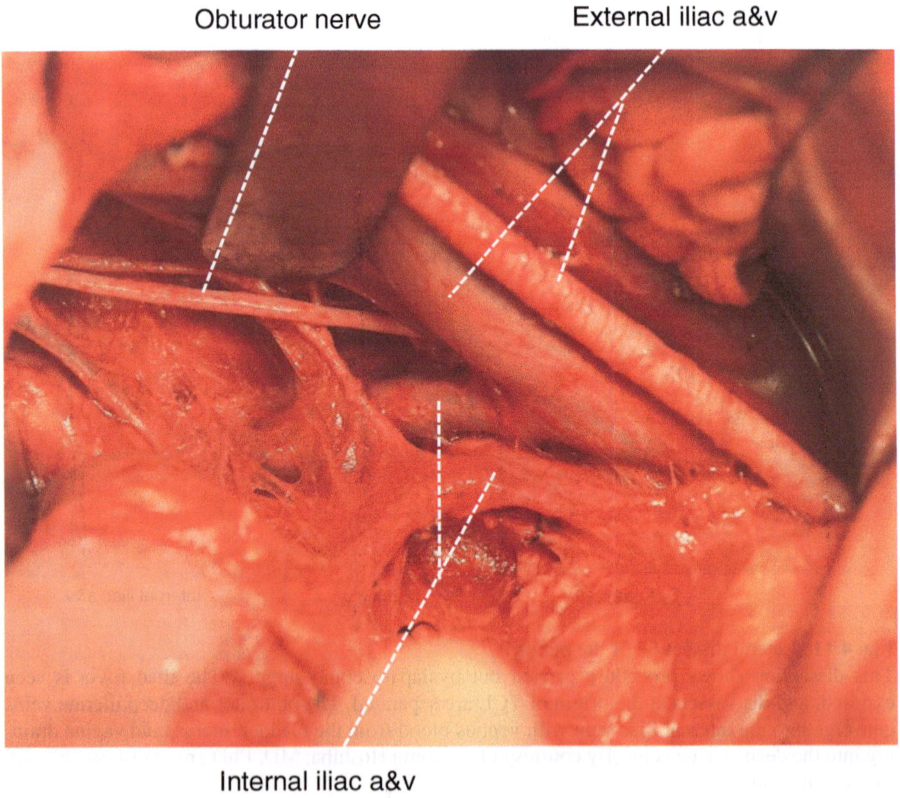

Fig. 4.13 Iliac vascular triangle
This photograph shows the venous triangle viewed from the medial aspect and the arterial triangle before clearance. This indicates that the internal iliac artery and external iliac vein are almost on the same level

trunk of the internal iliac vein and its branches such as the superior gluteal vein. It is also necessary to know that the internal iliac artery is on the same level as the external iliac vein, and after branching from the umbilical artery, it descends perpendicularly together with the internal iliac vein in the direction of S2 and S3 (Figs. 3.9 and 4.15).

The reason why repairing damage to the internal iliac vein presents difficulties lies not only at its branching point but also at its periphery. Fortunately, encounters with lymph node metastases in this area are rare, and the distribution of sentinel nodes is also low.

1.7.6 Clearance of the Common Iliac Lymph Nodes

This manipulation involves clearance of the lymph nodes of the external iliac vessels extending cranially (Figs. 3.10 and 4.16). Although this is generally the last step to be carried out in the procedure, the approach may need to be adjusted as required. Dealing perfectly with the posterior trunks of the internal iliac vessels is challenging (Fig. 3.9) and requires flexibility and adaptation in some cases.

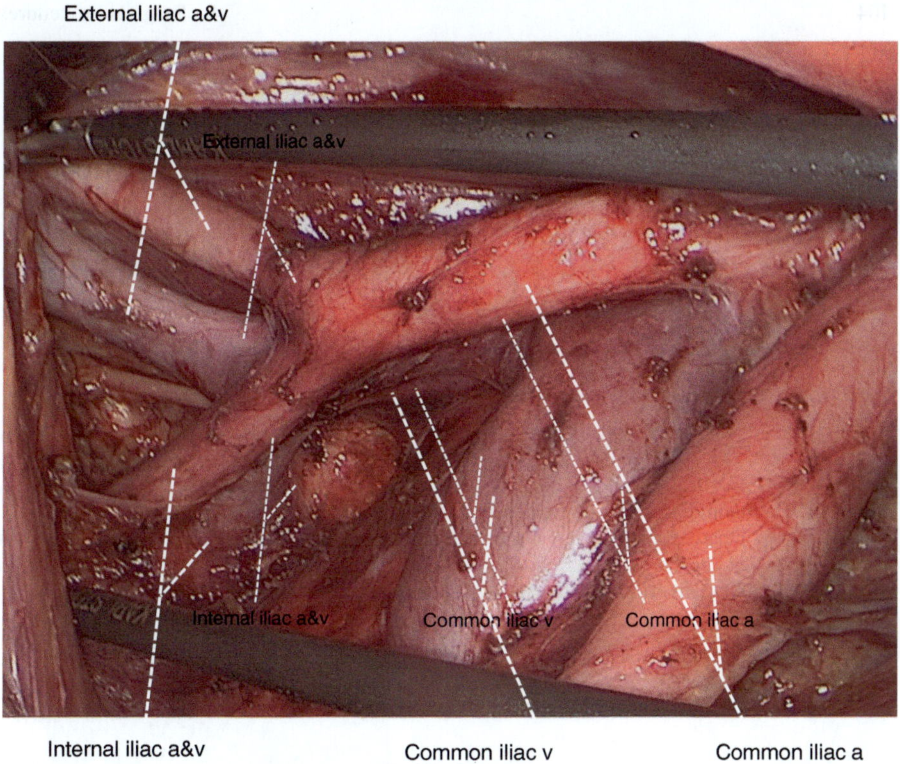

Fig. 4.14 Clearance of the triangles of the iliac vessels
Laparoscopic surgery is far more suitable and safer for clearance of the posterior aspect of the triangles of the iliac vessels. (By courtesy of Tsutomu Hoshiba, MD, PhD)

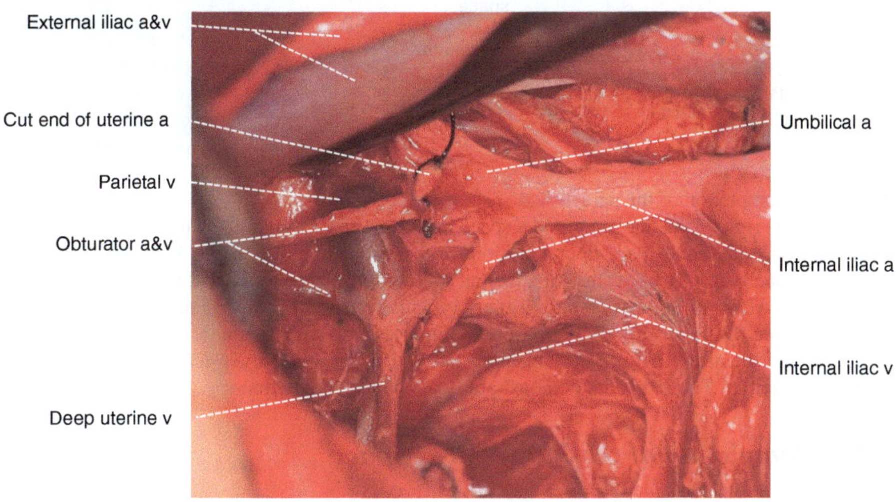

Fig. 4.15 Origin of the transverse cervical ligament and exposed anterior trunks of the internal iliac vessels
A photograph taken from the medial aspect of the right pelvic cavity. Here, the anterior trunk of the internal iliac artery gives off branches to the umbilical, uterine (resected), and obturator arteries before coursing toward the sacrum. The anterior trunk of the internal iliac vein consists of the deep uterine and obturator veins and a large parietal branch, amalgamating to form a single vessel

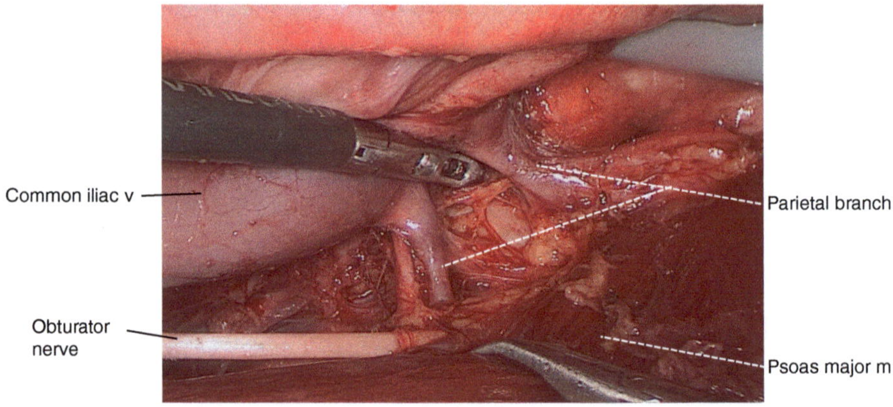

Fig. 4.16 Common iliac vein and psoas major muscle
Carried out by laparoscopic surgery, the posterior trunk of the internal iliac vein and numerous parietal branches can be seen to drain into the common iliac vein. (By courtesy of Tsutomu Hoshiba, MD, PhD., my most capable and trustworthy colleague)

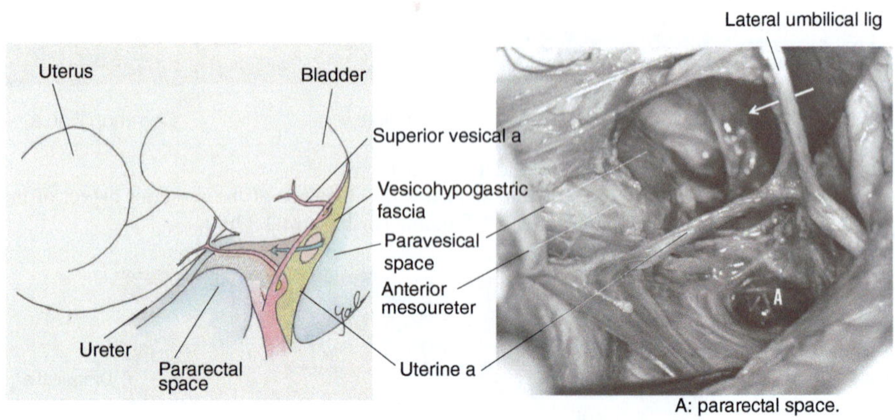

Fig. 4.17 Completion of the paravesical space
Shown on the right panel, the paravesical space must first be excavated so as to be positioned right in front of the pararectal space in preparation for this procedure to separate TCL. To accomplish this, this space is further excavated in a medial direction from the retroperitoneal space indicated by an arrow. After pulling up the umbilical artery and creating a window in the vesicohypogastric fascia between the superior vesical and uterine arteries, the areolar connective tissue is excised along the uterine artery between the bladder and uterus, and the paravesical space is excavated down to the ureter. The left panel demonstrates explanatory illustration

1.8 Completion of the Paravesical Space

This procedure involves excision of the anterior fascia of the lateral TCL that is revealed during exploratory excavation of the paravesical space and the latter's expansion medially by breaking through the vesicohypogastric fascia. This excavation is carried out until just lateral to the ureter (Fig. 4.17), for only then can the anterior mesoureter be visualized, enabling comparison of the paravesical space to

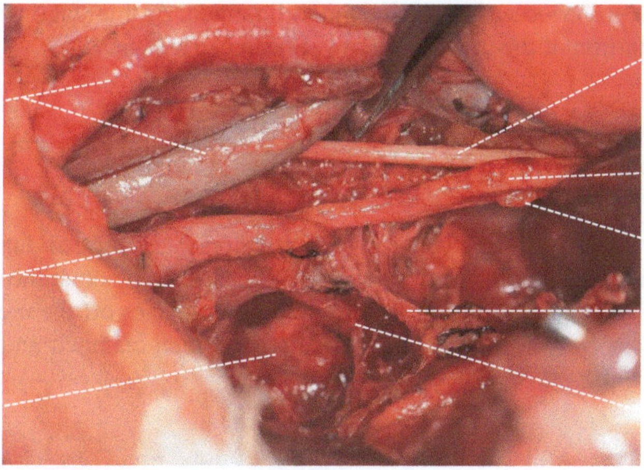

Fig. 4.18 Separation of the deep uterine vein
Shown is the left pelvic wall viewed from the medial aspect. This procedure brings us close to the completion of excision of TCL. This figure shows the outlines of the deep uterine vein and inferior vesical vessels almost exposed, followed by suction to further clear the site of origin of the excised TCL

the fourth space. This technique to create a window involves, first, lifting the lateral umbilical ligament between the uterine and superior vesical arteries within the vesicohypogastric fascia (left side in Fig. 4.17). Then, the loose connective tissue between the uterine artery and bladder is separated to create a space, reaching to the ureter/anterior mesoureter. During this process, the use of a suction apparatus and/or CUSA can be convenient for the removal of the anterior fascia of TCL and fatty-areolar connective tissue. Simultaneously, clearance around the uterine artery and deep uterine vein is carried out as part of the posterior fascia manipulation, completing approximately 80% of the separation (Fig. 4.18). It is worth noting that branches from the uterine artery sometimes include those from the superior vesical and/or vaginal arteries. In the vicinity of the anterior mesoureter, the use of CUSA is contraindicated. Caution regarding the use of CUSA has previously been stated.

1.9 Completion of Latzko's Paravesical Space

The main focus of this procedure is expansion of Latzko's pararectal space and removal of the vascular sheath of the internal iliac vessels and posterior fascia of TCL from their respective tissues. While carrying out excision of the posterior fascia and areolar connective tissue using manual and suction dissection or CUSA, clear the area around the uterine artery and deep uterine vein synchronized with excision of the anterior fascia (Fig. 4.18), not exposing the sacral plexus, fascia of the piriformis muscle, and pelvic splanchnic nerve (Fig. 3.7). By this manipulation, the detached portion of the vascular sheath of the internal iliac vessels and posterior fascia of TCL are pushed to the medial aspect of the pararectal space, bonding with the back of the posterior leaf of uterine broad ligament. At this stage, separation of the posterior portion of the ureter has not yet been carried out.

1.10 Severance of the Denuded Uterine Artery

The uterine artery at the upper edge of TCL has already been freed during excavation of the paravesical and pararectal spaces. This artery is, sometimes, accompanied by the superficial uterine vein, and frequently branches off the ureteral artery that is usually not preserved. The uterine artery is then clamped and severed at its origin.

1.11 Separation and Ligature of the Deep Uterine Vein

The deep uterine vein flows into the internal iliac vein at approximately the same location as the obturator vein. The area around this confluence is thoroughly cleared using liposuction or CUSA (Figs. 4.11 and 4.18). The separated deep uterine vein used as a marker is only ligated and not excised.

1.12 Excavation of Okabayashi's Pararectal Space and Separation of the Ureter/Posterior Mesoureter

Here, Latzko's excavated pararectal space shows the posterior portion of the ureter adhering to the posterior leaf of the uterine broad ligament. Okabayashi's pararectal space is created between the serosa of the posterior leaf of the uterine broad ligament and underlying subserous fascia. While pulling the posterior leaf of the uterine broad ligament as shown in Fig. 4.19a, an incision is made posteriorly in the subserous fascial lining, separating it from the subserous layer and ureter, thereby creating a space (panel (**b**) of Fig. 4.19).

Figure 4.20 shows an intraoperative finding of Okabayashi's pararectal space excavated between the posterior leaf, or *serosa*, of the uterine broad ligament and ureter/posterior mesoureter. Through this procedure, the posterior leaf, or *serosa*, of the uterine broad ligament is completely separated.

Figure 4.21 depicts a simulated dissection of Okabayashi's pararectal space on a fresh cadaver. In panel (**a**), following dissection, the posterior mesoureter is seen merging with the ureter, along with the hypogastric nerve passing within it. Panel (**b**) shows Okabayashi's pararectal space excavated down to the pelvic floor, with the hypogastric nerve, pelvic splanchnic nerves, and inferior hypogastric plexus exposed. This is frequently observed in classical RH with the removal of the lateral rectal ligament. However, in NSRH, the excavation is halted at a level just above, or *ventral to*, the hypogastric nerve. In the anatomic dissection shown in Fig. 3.7, the deep uterine

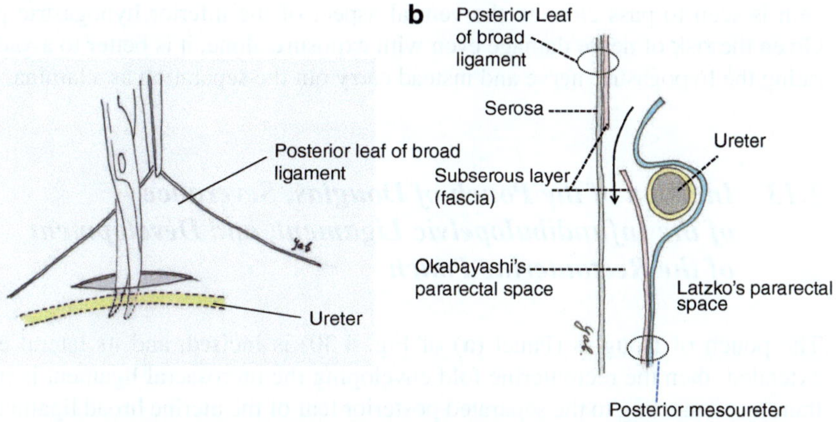

Fig. 4.19 Schematic illustrations demonstrating the creation of Okabayashi's pararectal space
Panel (**a**) demonstrates a shallow incision made on the upper part, or *ventral aspect*, of the posterior leaf of the uterine broad ligament to which the ureter attaches
Panel (**b**): Okabayashi's pararectal space is created by entering between the posterior leaf of the uterine broad ligament, or *serosa*, and underlying subserous fascia, thereby separating them

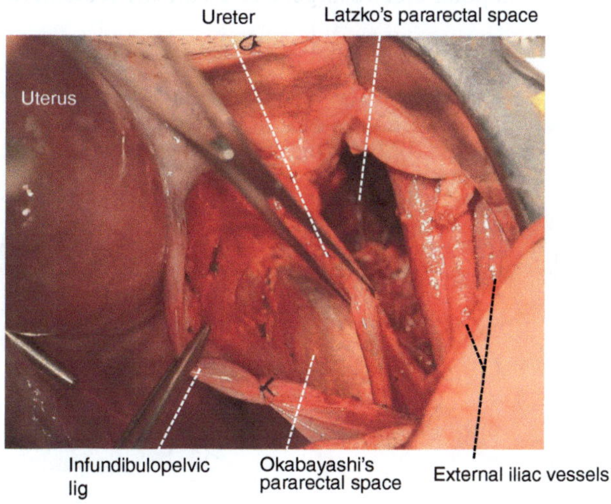

Fig. 4.20 Intraoperative findings from creation of Okabayashi's pararectal space
This photograph shows a bird's-eye view of the right pelvic cavity, and the bottom indicates the cranial aspect. Okabayashi's pararectal space is excavated between the ureter, which is seen lifted with Allis forceps, and the posterior leaf of the uterine broad ligament that is grasped with forceps. Latzko's pararectal space is developed on the lateral aspect of the ureter with both spaces being separated by the posterior mesoureter

vein is seen to pass close to the ventral aspect of the inferior hypogastric plexus. Given the risk of nerve damage even with exposure alone, it is better to avoid separating the hypogastric nerve and instead carry out the separation as a lamina.

1.13 Incision of the Pouch of Douglas, Severance of the Infundibulopelvic Ligament, and Development of the Rectouterine Pouch

The pouch of Douglas (Panel (**a**) of Fig. 4.30) is incised, and its lateral edge is extended, then the rectouterine fold enveloping the uterosacral ligament is incised, thereby connecting to the separated posterior leaf of the uterine broad ligament. The incised posterior leaf, which has been separated by the creation of Okabayshi's pararectal space, connects to the infundibulopelvic ligament and, while paying close attention to the ureter, it is then excised (a red double-headed dashed arrow in panel (**a**) of Fig. 4.21). Next, a rectal hook is inserted into the posterior vaginal wall and, while being pulled, the anterior wall of the sigmoid colon is pressed with the fingers, creating tension in the intervening loose connective tissue. This tissue is then incised using monopolar electrosurgery to create the rectouterine pouch. This

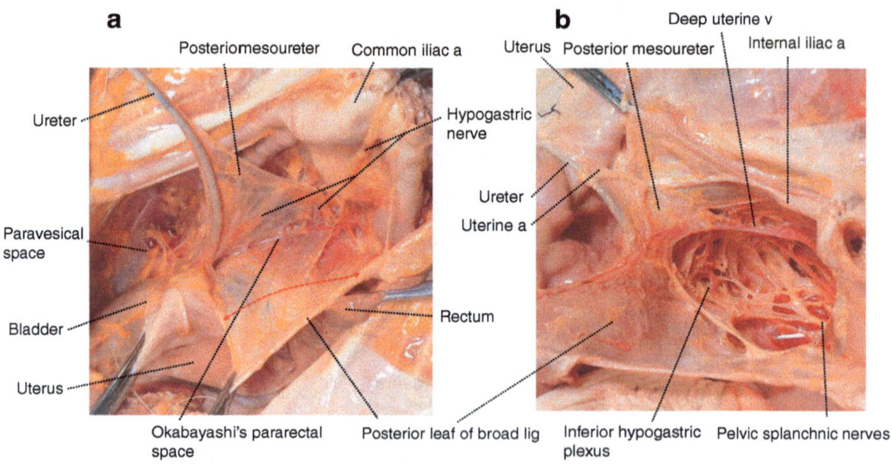

Fig. 4.21 Posterior mesoureter and Okabayashi's pararectal space
Panel (**a**) represents the anatomic findings of the right pelvic cavity on a fresh cadaver. The uterus is being pulled caudally or *left*. This photograph shows the fascia underlying the posterior leaf of the uterine broad ligament being separated from the serosa of its ligament along with the ureter and hypogastric nerve so as to isolate the posterior mesoureter. If this excision is further extended to the dorsal aspect, Okabayashi's pararectal space will be developed. (Reproduced from Yabuki et al. 2005)
Panel (**b**) represents the separated pelvic autonomic nerve. Okabayashi's pararectal space is seen excavated down to the pelvic floor, exposing the inferior hypogastric plexus and pelvic splanchnic nerves. However, in an actual RH, exposure of these nerves is not carried out

procedure results in the separation of the rectouterine ligament between the recto-uterine pouch and Okabayashi's pararectal space (Fig. 4.23).

1.14 Fenestration of the Posterior Mesoureter

The extent of excision of the posterior mesoureter has the following boundaries: on the ventral aspect, or the upper end, excision extends to the lower edge of the ureter capsule, while preserving as much as possible the ureteral branches of the uterine and internal iliac arteries. On the dorsal aspect, or the lower end, it reaches to the upper edge of the hypogastric nerve. On the caudal aspect, it extends to the posterior aspect of TCL and, on the cranial aspect, it reaches to the site of detachment of the infundibulopelvic ligament. Through this created window, as seen in Fig. 4.22, parietal vascular structures and the deep uterine vein can be observed.

Detachment and separation of the deep uterine vein from the underlying tissues are best carried out in a direction shown in Fig. 4.23. This approach, often referred to as "lifting off," allows for more precision and reduces the risk of damage while pulling the vein upward.

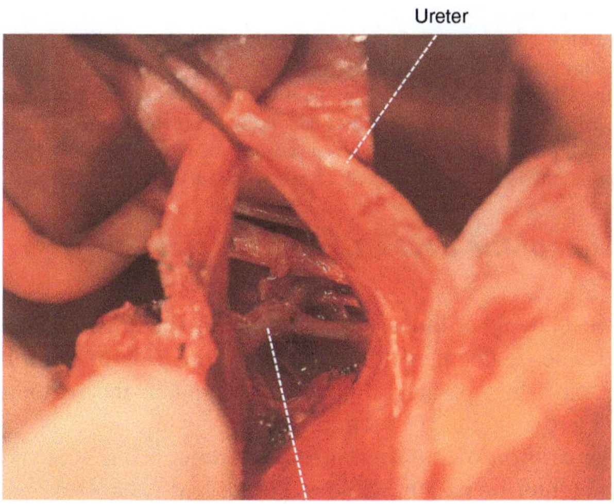

Fig. 4.22 Excision of the posterior mesoureter by creation of a window
This photograph is from a medial aspect of the right pelvic cavity. Shown is the right cranial aspect. A window is created in the posterior mesoureter followed by the creation of Latzko's and Okabayashi's pararectal spaces. Then the sheath of the internal iliac vessels, posterior fascia of TCL, and fascia of the posterior leaf of the uterine broad ligament, all of which attach to the meso-ureter, are simultaneously excised. Observed through this window of the ureteric plate is the deep uterine vein ascending toward the uterus

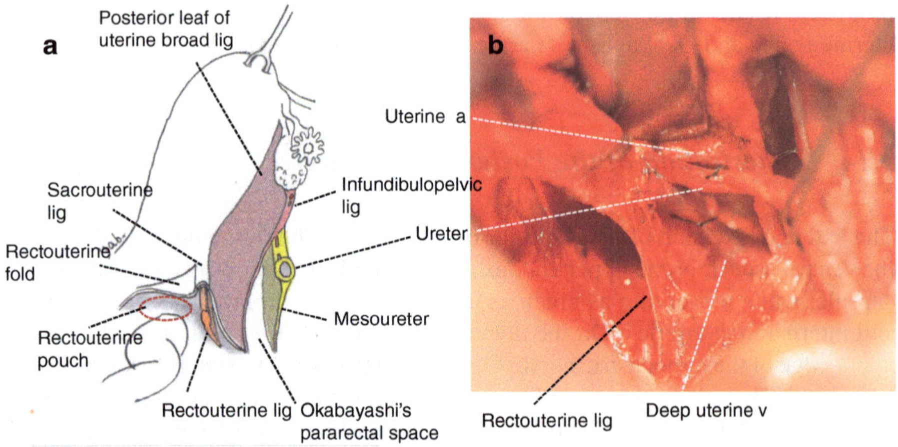

Fig. 4.23 The sequence of the separated rectouterine ligament, uterine artery, ureter, and deep uterine vein
Panel (**a**) represents a schematic illustration centered around the peritoneum on the posterior aspect of the uterus. The peritoneum consists of serosa and subserous tissue. Okabayashi's pararectal space advocated by the author corresponds to a space resulting from dividing the posterior leaf of the uterine broad ligament into two. Moreover, this illustration is based on the fact that the uterosacral ligament corresponds to the tip of the rectouterine ligament covered by peritoneum that is termed as a plica or fold
Panel (**b**): Cranial view showing the right parametrial tissue representing separation of the rectouterine ligament thinned from the rectouterine pouch and Okabayashi's pararectal space. By strongly pulling the uterus to the left in a cranioventral direction, the uterine artery is seen climbing over the ureter, while the deep uterine vein ascends along the rectouterine ligament and slips under the ureter, reaching the uterus. From these observations, the concept of a common pedicle for the uterosacral ligament and TCL can be refuted. (Reproduced from Yabuki 2023)

1.15 Excision of the Rectouterine Ligament

In this area almost devoid of blood vessels, by using the fingers or a suction apparatus, the rectouterine ligament is thinned from a direction of both the rectouterine pouch and Okabayashi's pararectal space, resulting in the rectouterine ligament being separated to the side of the rectum.

Following separation of the rectouterine ligament, one leaf of the forceps is placed in the rectouterine pouch, while the other leaf is hooked into Okabayashi's pararectal space followed by clamping and excision of the ligament. However, it is important to keep the following scenario in mind when planning the surgery, for, through this well-developed pararectal space, the sequence of the rectouterine ligament, uterine artery, ureter, and deep uterine vein can be appreciated (Fig. 4.23).

1.16 Mobilization of the Bladder and Development of the Vesicouterine Pouch

This detachment is carried out meticulously up to the supravaginal septum until the connection between the bladder and vagina becomes somewhat dense, and, then laterally, until the bladder pillar becomes visible. Similar to the detachment of the rectouterine pouch, sharp excision of the loose connective tissue between the bladder and uterine cervix is carried out, while avoiding any rubbing with gauze or similar materials.

1.17 Excision of the Vesicouterine Ligament (VUL)

The author classifies Okabayashi's vesicouterine ligament into the following three layers: The first layer consists of the so-called fascial true ligament, or *bladder pillar*, connecting the bladder and uterus; the second layer comprises the areolar connective tissue between the bladder pillar and ureter; and the third layer involves the neurovascular bundle, or *anterior mesoureter*, hanging from the ureter (panels (**b**) of Figs. 4.28 and 4.29). These three layers are processed as follows:

1.17.1 Processing of the Second Layer, or Creation of the Fourth Space

Here will be described Okabayashi's paravaginal space or the author's fourth space as excavated in the areolar connective tissue indicated by an ellipse in panel (**a**) of Fig. 3.14. According to Okabayashi's surgical technique, panel (**a**) of Fig. 4.24 shows the separated anterior layer, or *ureteric roof*, following creation of the ureteric tunnel from the medial aspect of the ureter, which is then excised to expose Okabayashi's paravaginal space.

Panel (**b**) of Fig. 4.24 shows the paravaginal space created by Dr. Tomoyasu Kato at the Department of Gynecology, National Cancer Center Hospital, Japan, following the Okabayashi procedure.

Panel (**a**) of Fig. 4.25 shows an open abdominal RH and panel (**b**) the fourth space that has been excavated in laparoscopic RH by the use of "open-air" excavation. This procedure was carried out under direct visualization from the tip of the Kelly clamp, which ensures a high level of safety.

The author will describe in this section the technique for excavating the fourth space. But first, let's look at panel (**a**) of Fig. 4.26 that illustrates the excavation site for the fourth space. Although not intentionally drawn by P&A to depict the fourth space, a white x in panel (**b**) coincides with the excavation site for the fourth space in panel (**a**) of Fig. 4.26, which corresponds to the location of the ellipse in panel (**b**) of Fig. 3.13 and panel (**a**) of Fig. 3.14. This demonstrates the excellent observational skills of P&A.

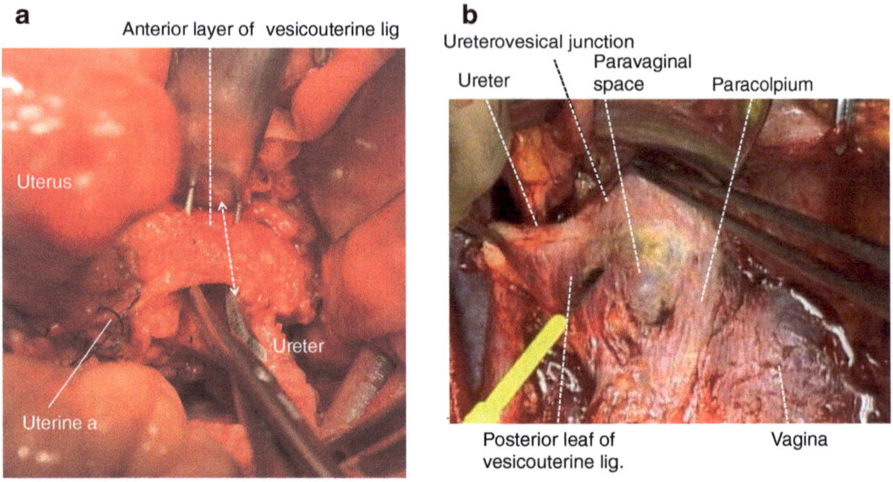

Fig. 4.24 Intraoperative images of the anterior layer of the vesicouterine ligament separated in the Okabayashi procedure and exposure of the paravaginal space
Panel (**a**): The author created the ureteral tunnel to separate the anterior layer of the vesicouterine ligament
Panel (**b**) was provided by Dr. Tomoyasu Kato of the Department of Gynecology, National Cancer Center Hospital, Japan. This shows where the anterior layer is excised, exposing the paravaginal space

To continue with surgical techniques for excavation, it should be noted that the bladder edge between the bladder pillar and ureterovesical junction is frequently unclear. In such a case, aim at a point approximately 2 cm from the cranial aspect of the ureterovesical junction, then gently tease the loose connective tissue between the bladder pillar and ureter from a cranial to caudal direction using the tip of the second finger or tip of Cooper scissors. Then, place a small hook retractor and lightly pull it caudally (white arrow in panel (**b**) of Fig. 4.26).

Next, as shown in panel (**a**) of Fig. 4.27, the bladder pillar is grasped with Allis forceps, and the tip of a Kelly clamp is placed approximately 1.5 to 2 cm cranially to the edge of the bladder that is held by a muscle hook retractor. Then, gently open and close the Kelly clamp while excavating perpendicularly in a dorsal direction. To avoid damaging the blood vessels running along the sidewall of the uterine cervix, be mindful of them as you excavate approximately 3 cm deeper than the ureter. Occasionally, one may encounter vessels crossing the space, but they are easily

Fig. 4.25 Intraoperative observation of the fourth space exposed by open excavation and laparoscopic surgery
Panel (**a**) represents development of the fourth space at the stage when the inserted Kelly forceps are open with the ureter already freed with hardly any blood vessels visible
Panel (**b**) represents the fourth space dissected during laparoscopic surgery. The bladder pillar is seen being pulled cranially to prevent displacement of the bladder. (By courtesy of Tsutomu Hoshiba, MD, PhD., my most capable and trustworthy colleague)

a

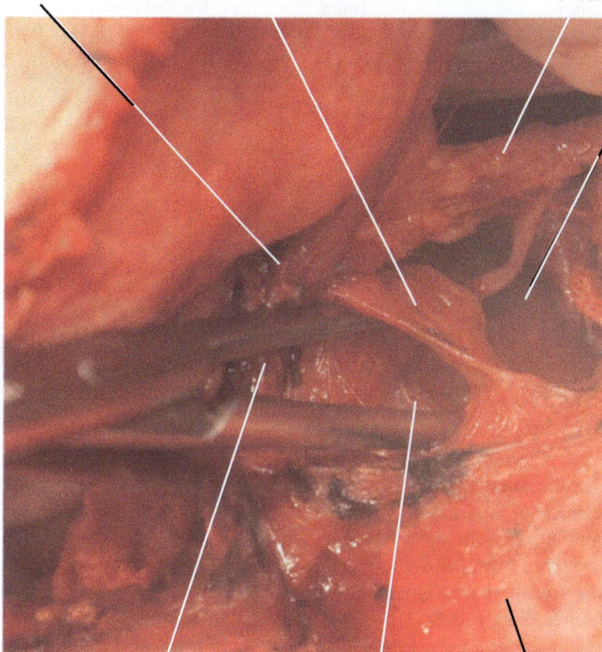
Paravesical space
Bladder
Anterior mesoureter
Ureter
Deep uterine v
Fourth space
Cervix

b

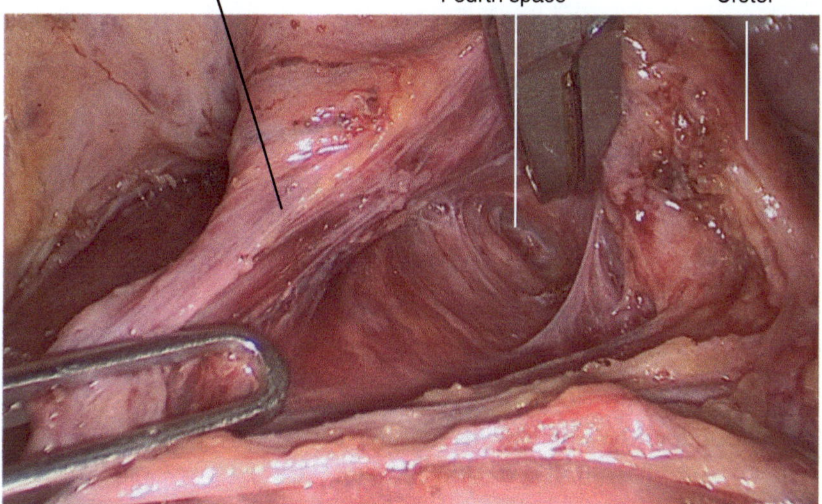
Bladder pillar
Fourth space
Ureter

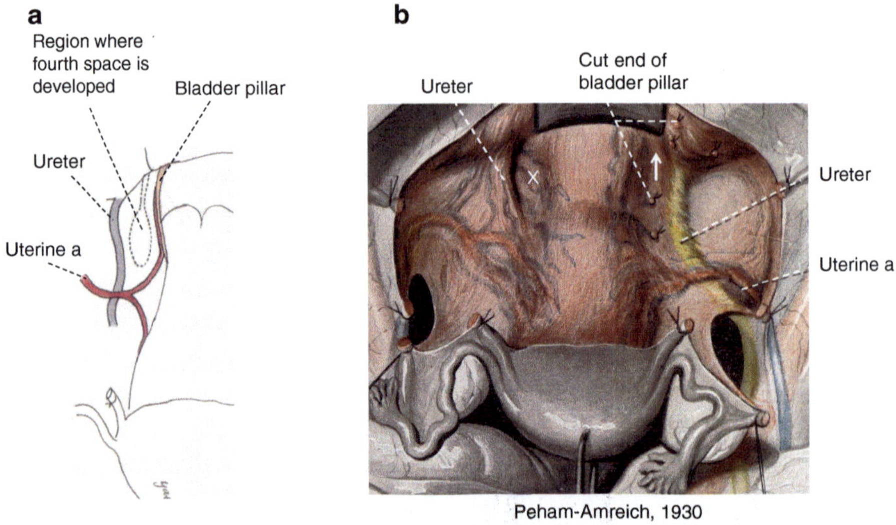

Fig. 4.26 Location for the excavation of the fourth space
Panel (**a**) shows excavation of the fourth space carried out in the areolar connective tissue between the ureter and the lateral edge of the uterine cervix
Panel (**b**): A figure borrowed from P&A's surgical manual has been marked with an X showing the excavation site for the fourth space. This area corresponds to Savage/Kocks' CL. (Reproduced from Peham and Amreich 1930, Fig. 203, p. 358)

identified and do not cause hemorrhaging. Then, in a cranial direction, expand the space as far as the ureteric-uterine artery junction (panel (**b**)). Finally, excavate a tunnel between the fourth space and Okabayashi's pararectal space to remove the roof (yellow double-headed arrow). This exposes the middle portion of the ureter. Thus, between the excavated fourth space and paravesical space is the separated ureter/anterior mesoureter with the fourth space not being excavated down to the pelvic floor.

1.17.2 Severance of the So-Called Vesicouterine Ligament, or Bladder Pillar

The bladder pillar (panel (**a**) of Fig. 4.27) that appears between the vesicouterine pouch and fourth space is clamped with forceps and excised. To avoid hemorrhaging, care should be taken not to touch the descending branches of the uterine vessels.

1.17.3 Processing of the Anterior Mesoureter and Nerve-Sparing Procedure

The final step in handling the vesicouterine ligament involves the severance of the anterior mesoureter. However, it is important to note that not all of the tissues seen separated in Fig. 3.18 are excised.

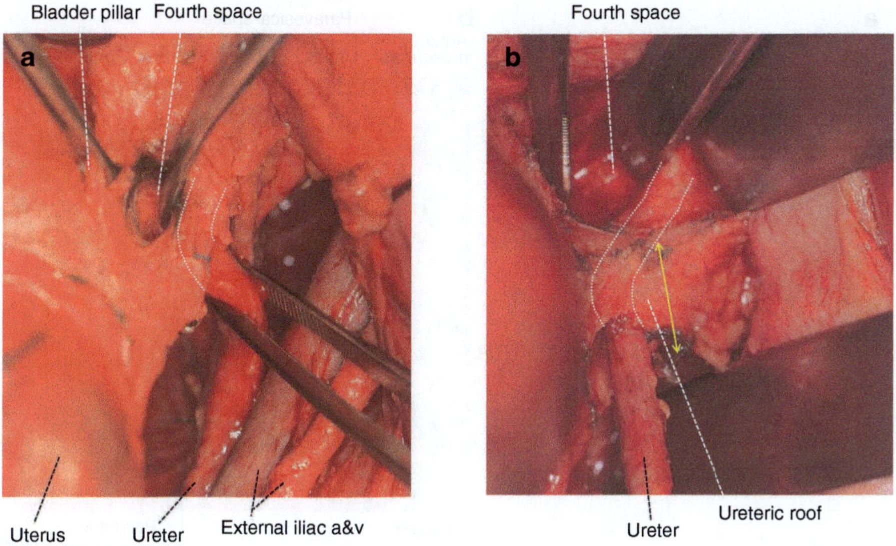

Fig. 4.27 Intraoperative findings during excavation of the fourth space
Panel (**a**): Excavation of the fourth space is carried out by grasping and pulling up the bladder pillar with Allis forceps, at the same time, advancing the tip of the Kelly forceps perpendicular to the loose connective tissue between the ureter and uterine cervix, lightly opening and closing as progressing deeper. This space is filled with less vascular-areolar connective tissue
Panel (**b**): The fourth space is carefully expanded using Kelly forceps, Cooper scissors, and the spring-opening mechanism of Nélaton's forceps with the roof of the ureteric tunnel beginning to appear between the fourth space and Okabayashi's pararectal space. A tunnel is excavated from this fourth space to Okabayashi's pararectal space, and the roof is severed (yellow double arrow)

The fourth space has now been excavated, and at this point of the manipulation shown in panel (**b**) of Fig. 4.27, the mid-portion of the ureter can be seen exposed and free, and finally, the separation of the anterior portion of the ureter is carried out. As the schematic illustration shows in panel (**a**) of Fig. 4.28, the ureter is gently detached from the anterior mesoureter by rolling it upward using Cooper scissors. Once it is exposed, Kelly clamp is inserted just before the ureterovesical junction, and, in panel (**b**) of Fig. 4.28, the tip is seen entering into the paravesical space. This is followed by separation of the anterior portion of the ureter and anterior mesoureter along the yellow dashed line, releasing the ureter entirely up to the suspensory ligament.

Panel (**a**) of Fig. 4.29 depicts the anterior mesoureter freed after the separation of the ureter. This bundle connects the bladder and SS, and the blood vessels, or *superior vesical vein*, connecting the bladder and deep uterine vein appear transparent through it. The forceps are seen passed between the superior vesical vein and vesical nerve branches. If portrayed in a histological tissue image as in panel (**b**), this area would be represented by a double-headed red arrow drawn from the fourth space toward the paravesical space.

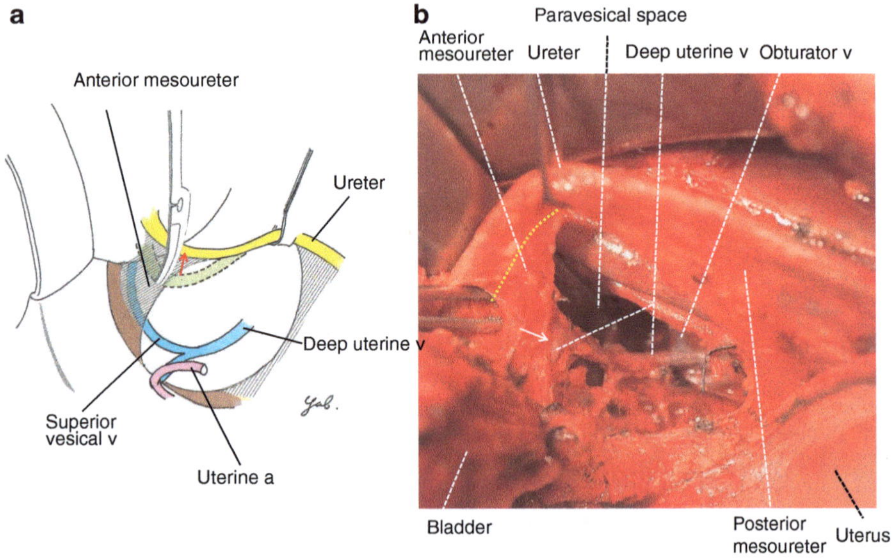

Fig. 4.28 Separation of the ureter and handling of the anterior mesoureter
Panel (**a**): This schematic illustration shows the procedure before separation of the ureter. The ureter is gently isolated upward, or toward the ventral aspect, from the mesoureter so as to expose the ureterovesical junction (red arrow). This maneuver is called "ureter rolling"
Panel (**b**): This procedure involves puncturing the paravesical space with Kelly forceps near the ureterovesical junction. Then, to separate the ureter and the anterior mesoureter, severe the space between them at the yellow dashed line shown on the figure. (Reproduced from Yabuki et al. 2000)

Figure 4.30 illustrates the surgical procedure in its final stage. Panel (**a**) depicts, together with the strongly pulled uterus, the reduced rectouterine ligament and the separated deep uterine vein with the faintly visible superior vesical vein (white arrow) merging into it. Panel (**b**) provides a bird's-eye view of the deep uterine vein and superior vesical vein. As shown in panels (**a**) and (**b**), the process of pulling the uterus upward and an accurate observation from a cranial and superior perspective is crucial to the success of this surgery. Also, meticulous excavation of the paravesical and pararectal spaces is required.

Figure 3.20 depicts histological specimens and Fig. 3.21 dissected cadaver showing the vesical nerve branch running along the dorsal aspect of the superior vesical vein. Based on these findings, nerve-sparing surgery has been shown to be feasible with resection extending to the level of the deep uterine vein for SS and to the level of the superior vesical vein for the anterior mesoureter, and this approach was utilized in practice in 1996 (Yabuki et al. 1996).

Figure 4.31 depicts the vesical nerve branch passing along the dorsal aspect of the superior vesical vein. As mentioned regarding the hypogastric nerve, mere exposure of nerves delays postoperative recovery of bladder function. Exposure of nerves should be kept to a minimum and then only when absolutely necessary.

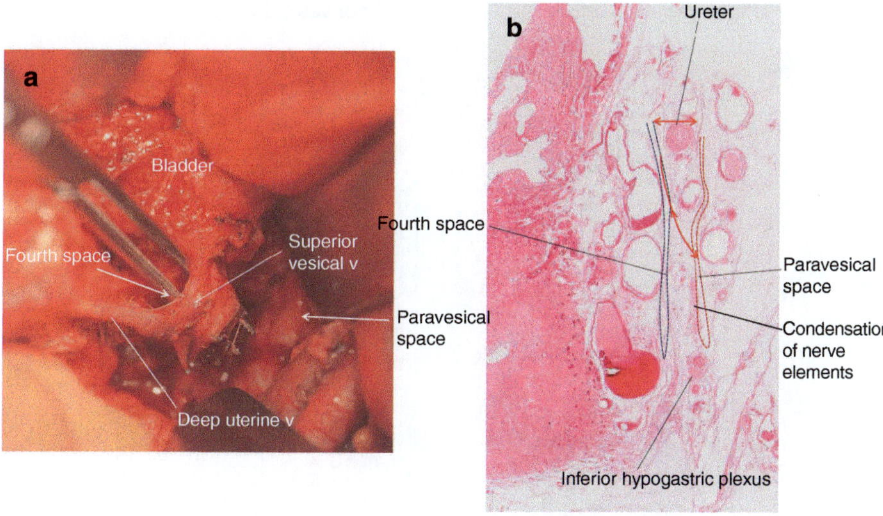

Fig. 4.29 Separation of the anterior mesoureter by the Okabayashi procedure
Panel (**a**) depicts a case from the time when the Okabayashi procedure was faithfully carried out. Kelly forceps is seen inserted from the fourth space perforating the inferior edge of the vesical nerve branch and exiting into the paravesical space, thereby separating the posterior leaf. Within the separated posterior leaf, the superior vesical vein passes and drains into the deep uterine vein. (Reproduced from Yabuki 2020)
Panel (**b**) illustrates the direction of insertion of the Kelly forceps penetrating from the fourth space through the anterior mesoureter and into the paravesical space, also demonstrated in panel (**b**) of Fig. 3.16. However, Okabayashi did not specify the range of excision of the anterior mesoureter

In cases of stage I cervical cancer, efforts should be made to separate only the veins without exposing the nerves once one has gained experience of the relationship between them. It should always be anticipated that there are often branches of the inferior vesical vein passing between the superior vesical vein and vesical nerve branches when separating the superior vesical vein. Using a suction apparatus and non-toothed forceps, excise it gently from the surrounding tissue to avoid damage to the vesical nerve branches. It is advisable to pass a suture through the slackest part of the connective tissue on the dorsal aspect of the superior vesical vein to lift it up (panel (**a**) of Fig. 4.33).

In cases of FIGO IB and IIA cervical cancer, the author has never encountered metastasis or infiltration into the anterior mesoureter. The possible reasons for this are presented in theories such as Höckel et al's hypothesis (2005) that the anterior mesoureter corresponds to the bladder mesentery, and also Kraima, et al's hypothesis (Kraima et al. 2014) regarding there is no lymphatic drainage pathway in the vesicouterine ligament.

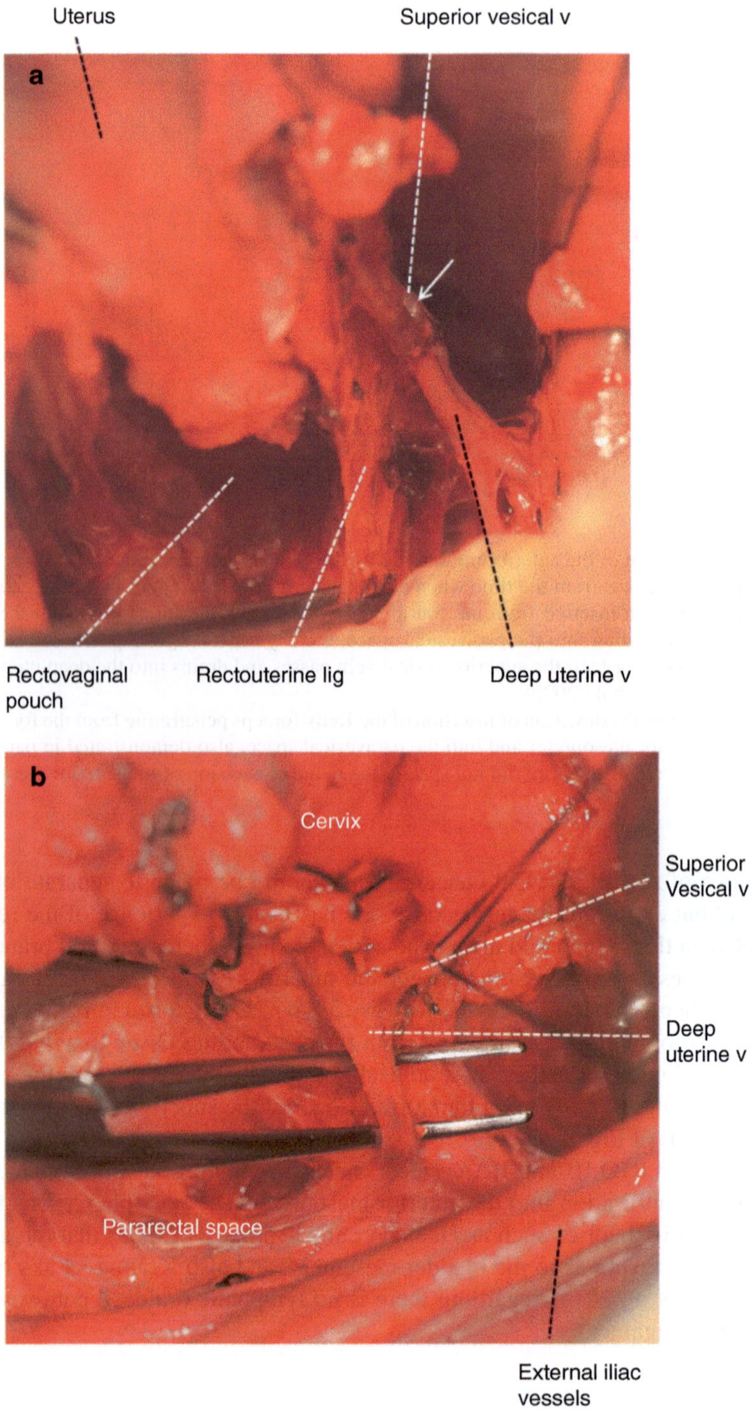
Uterus
Superior vesical v
a
Rectovaginal pouch
Rectouterine lig
Deep uterine v
b
Cervix
Superior Vesical v
Deep uterine v
Pararectal space
External iliac vessels

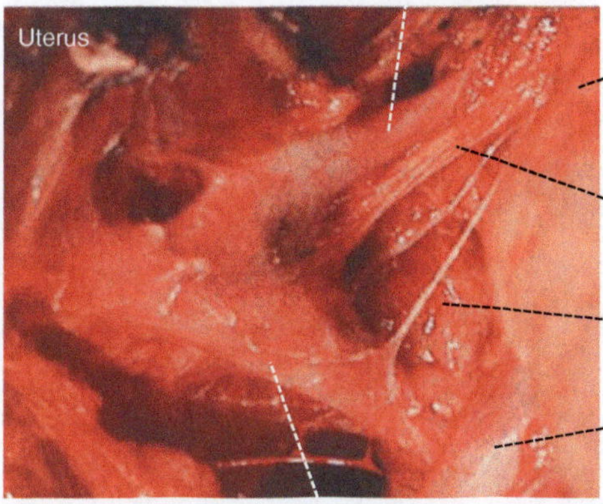

Fig. 4.31 Exposure of the superior vesical vein and vesical nerve branch
This image shows exposure of the superior vesical vein and vesical nerve branch by the development of the paravesical space. The deep uterine vein has not yet been fully separated, and the ureter is seen displaced laterally. The author's NSRH involves only the removal of the superior vesical vein while preserving the vesical nerves. (Reproduced from Yabuki 2020)

1.18 Excision of the Transverse Cervical Ligament (TCL)

This is the final step of the TCL procedure, in other words, the excision of the deep uterine vein. The preparatory procedure is almost completed as shown in Fig. 4.30. While also utilizing liposuction, it is essential to carefully confirm the clearance at the confluence of the deep uterine vein into the internal iliac vein (Fig. 4.32) and be aware that this area often includes the confluence of the obturator vein.

As mentioned, the first step is to expose the entire ventral aspect of the deep uterine vein, as illustrated in panel (**a**) of Fig. 4.33. Then, as depicted in Figs. 4.23 and 4.30, separate the deep uterine vein and underlying structures such as the inferior vesical vessels or the middle rectal artery from the direction of the pararectal space while visualizing the connection between them. Separation begins from the midportion of the vessel and extends toward both ends (panel (**a**) of Fig. 4.33). Panel (**b**) illustrates

Fig. 4.30 Separation of the deep uterine vein
As seen from the cranial aspect, panel (**a**) depicts an image of the right rectouterine ligament and deep uterine vein. The ureter is seen being displaced laterally. The photograph shows the deep uterine vein, separated by traction on the uterus, ascending toward it along the rectouterine ligament. Separation of the deep uterine vein from the underlying tissues in this direction is safer
Panel (**b**) depicts the separation by Kelly forceps of the deep uterine vein from the underlying tissues. In the upper right-hand corner, the superior vesical vein is seen draining from the bladder into the deep uterine vein. (Reproduced from Yabuki 2023)
The images depicted in the photographs of panels (**a**) and (**b**) suggest that the concept of the common pedicle does not seem to hold true from the viewpoint of clinical anatomy

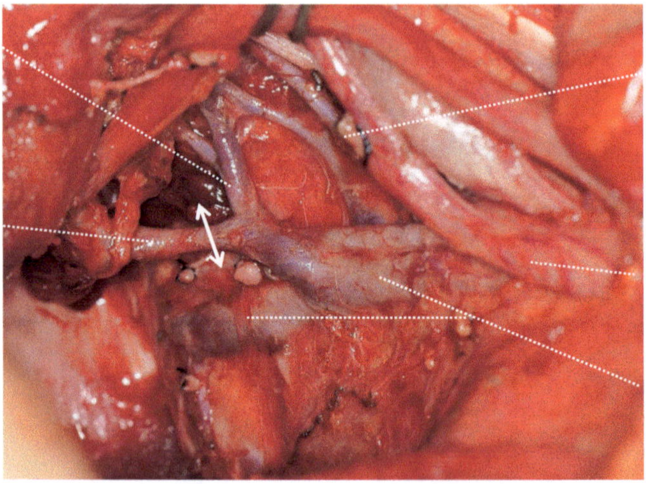

Fig. 4.32 Final inspection of the origin of TCL
Following pelvic lymphadenectomy, the origin of TCL is exposed and then thoroughly inspected. This is followed by its excision at the site shown by the double-headed arrow

the scene where the deep uterine vein that has been severed at the confluence of the internal iliac vein is being separated from the underlying structures while being pulled vertically. Sometimes, there is a confluence of veins indicated by the white arrow.

However, as seen in the cadaver in Fig. 3.12, the course of blood vessels in SS can be complex with intersections and anastomoses, making it difficult to identify and separate the vessels. In such cases, there is a risk of overlooking these anastomoses or communicating branches of the underlying vessels when using this method of vertically pulling the inner end thread of the deep uterine vein to detach it from the underlying structures (white arrow in panel (**b**) of Fig. 4.33). Separation from the inferior vesical vein can, in some cases, be particularly challenging. In cases where there are vascular intersections and anastomoses, especially involving veins, it is advisable not to force separation but rather meticulously expose and clear the surrounding tissue of fused vessels using a suction apparatus or, sometimes, CUSA. The recommended approach for the excision of the deep uterine vein

Fig. 4.33 Excision of the deep uterine vein
This is viewed from a left cranial aspect of the right pelvic cavity
Panel (**a**) shows the deep uterine vein separated from the underlying tissues using Kelly forceps, while the superior vesical vein is seen lifted with two silk threads
Panel (**b**): The superior vesical vein is severed at the side of the bladder, separating it up to its confluence with the deep uterine vein. Next, before its confluence with the internal iliac vein, the deep uterine vein is ligated at two points and severed in between. The ligature on the medial stump of the deep uterine vein is lifted, while excising any remaining attachments until it is sufficiently detached from the rectouterine ligament to reach the uterus

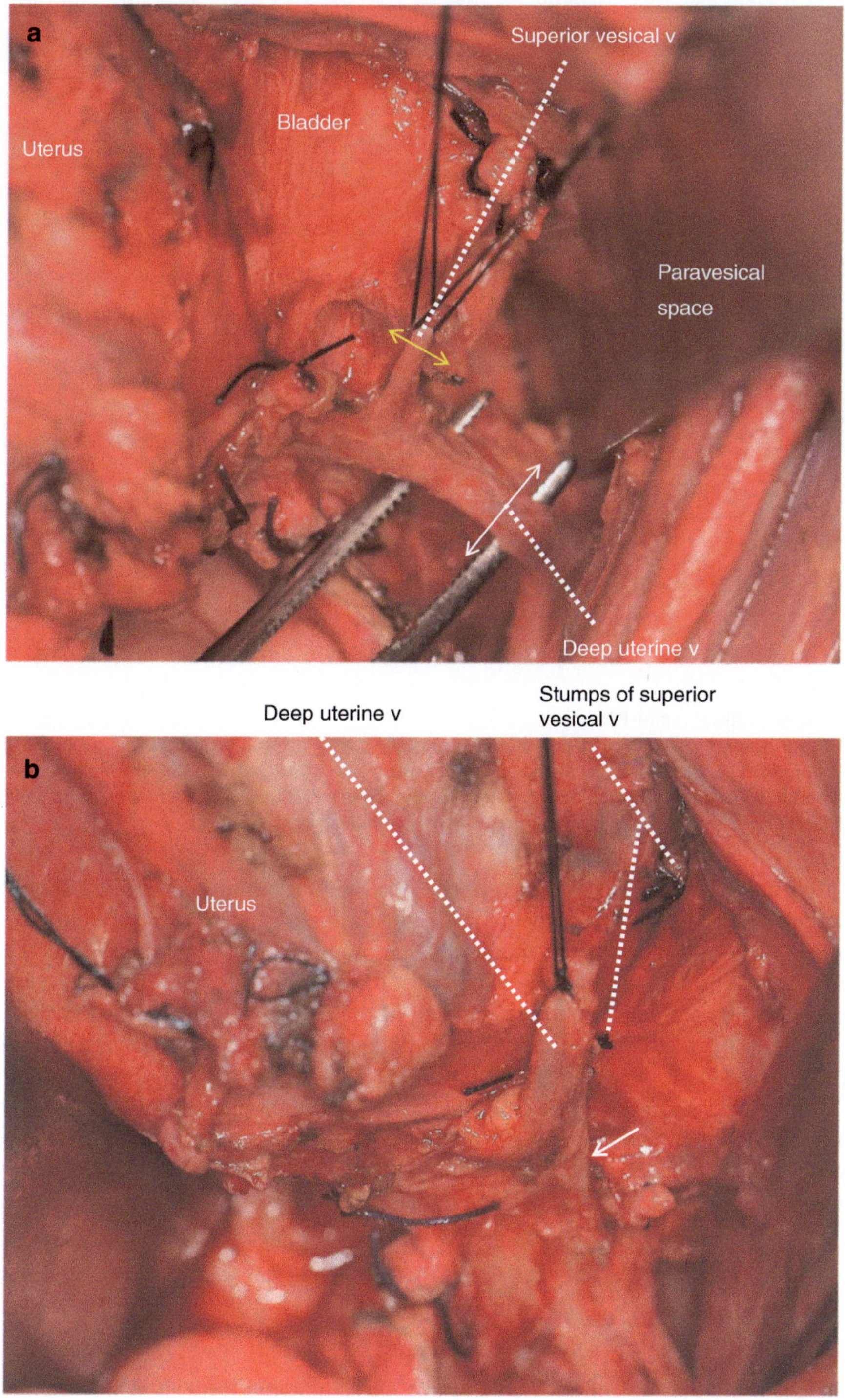
a
Superior vesical v
Bladder
Uterus
Paravesical
space
Deep uterine v
Deep uterine v
Stumps of superior
vesical v
b
Uterus

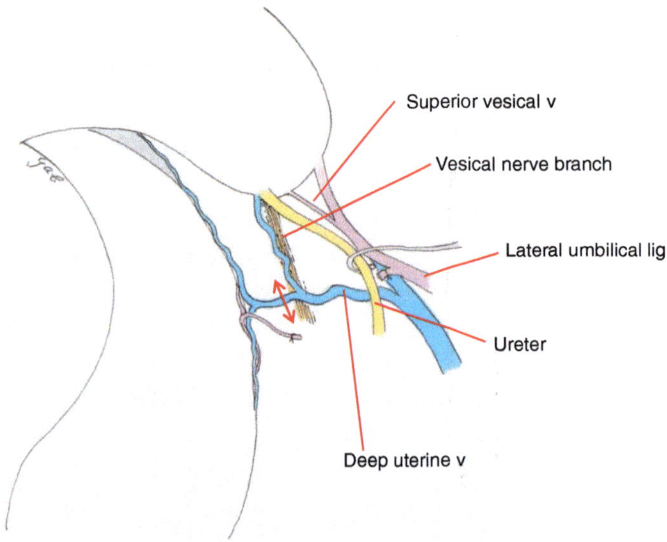

Fig. 4.34 Author's semi-RH
The fourth space is excavated, and the deep uterine vein is severed on the medial aspect of the mesoureter. Then, the paravesical and pararectal spaces are excavated, and the surrounding area is cleared including the origin of the deep uterine vein. However, the surgery becomes unexpectedly easier by not separating the deep uterine vein and its underlying tissues

is to remove it from the medial aspect of the confluent portion with the superior vesical vein (Fig. 4.34). With this method, the deep uterine vein is completely excised at its periphery from the confluence with the superior vesical vein. This technique, which involves the separation of the deep uterine vein from the medial aspect of the confluence to the attachment of the uterus followed by its severance/excision at the medial aspect of the mesoureter, is defined by the author as a semi-RH (Fig. 4.34).

Figure 4.35 shows completion of lateral manipulation in RH. The stumps of the excised deep uterine vein are seen lifted up, and the rectouterine/vaginal ligaments are to be excised along the line indicated by the yellow arrow. The white arrows indicate the passage of the pelvic autonomic nerve.

1.19 Paracolpectomy

The anatomic findings of SS including the lateral parametrium show that the vesicohypogastric fascia, TCL, and lateral rectal ligament form a single plate, as demonstrated in Figs. 3.7 and 4.36, which connects perpendicularly to the pelvic organs

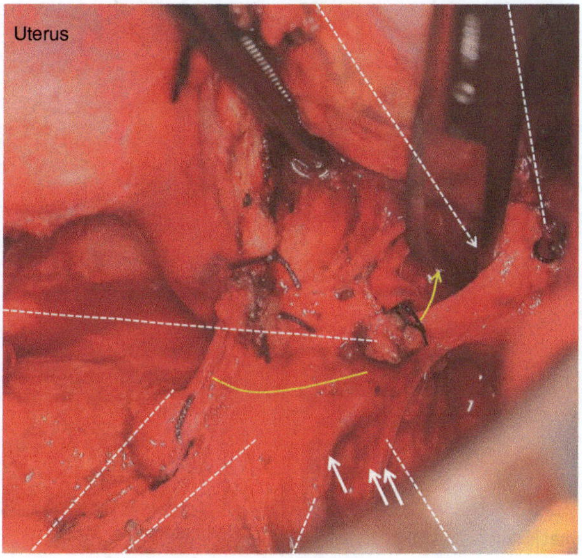

Fig. 4.35 The completion of nerve-sparing surgery
Here, the excavation of the fourth space, division and severance of the superior vesical vein/deep uterine vein, and manipulation of the anterior mesoureter have been completed with the passages of the hypogastric nerve and pelvic splanchnic nerve being preserved (white arrows). When lifting the overlapped stumps of the deep uterine vein and superior vesical vein, the dissection line (yellow arrow) for the rectovaginal ligament appears

and the pelvic sidewall by the transversal neurovascular bundle. In contrast, the paracolpium corresponds to a longitudinal neurovascular bundle (dashed white ellipse in Fig. 4.37) that passes between the vagina and tendinous arch of the pelvic fascia.

Figure 4.38 is a frontally sectioned histological image of the lateral ligament of the bladder, vagina, and rectum. The paracystium, paracolpium, and paraproctium run along the lateral border of their respective organs and connect to the pelvic sidewall via the tendinous arch of the pelvic fascia via the superior fascia of the pelvic diaphragm.

Parametrectomy is a method of perpendicularly dissecting TCL that has been separated by excavation of the paravesical and pararectal spaces (Figs. 2.12 and 2.18). In contrast, paracolpectomy involves horizontally detaching the paracolpium that has been exposed by extending the fourth space caudally (Figs. 3.27, 3.28 and 3.29). This excavated fourth space shown in Fig. 4.25 can be readily extended caudally as depicted in Fig. 4.39 and panel (**a**) of Fig. 4.40. By comparing the histological tissue images of panels (**b**) of Figs. 3.8 and 3.27 and 4.38, it can be understood that the dashed white line depicting the parametrium and dashed black line the paracolpium in Fig. 3.12 show the tissues are not of the same anatomic morphology.

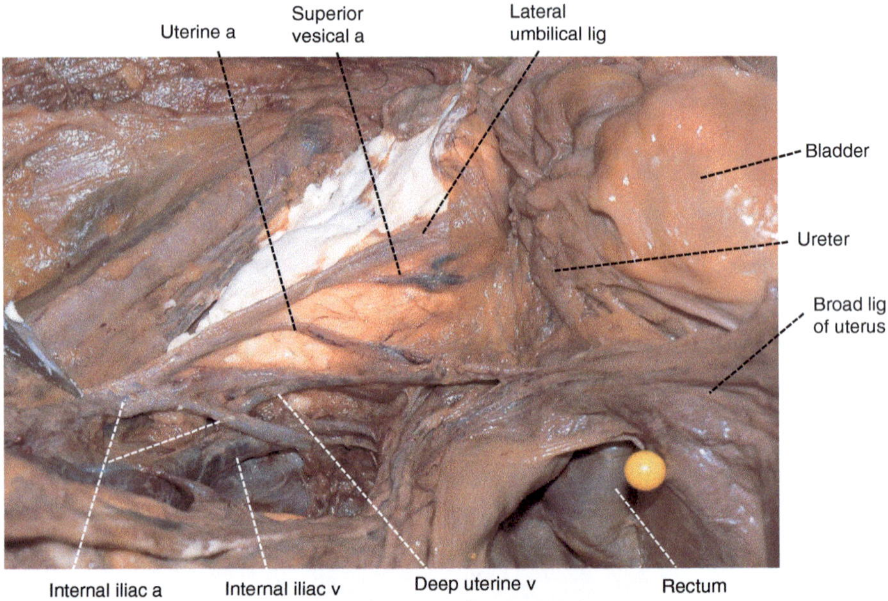

Fig. 4.36 Fixed cadaver dissection showing the posterior aspect of the supporting system as seen from Latzko's pararectal space
Seen here is the posterior aspect of SS dissected in the Latzko procedure. The area with the white packing represents the left paravesial space with the posterior fascia of SS having been excised, while the anterior fascia facing the paravesical space has been preserved with the vessels within SS separated. With the trunk of the internal iliac artery acting as the origin of the umbilical artery, superior vesical artery, uterine artery, deep uterine vein, middle rectal artery, and middle rectal vein; together, they form a single plate

Figure 4.40 illustrates the surgical separation of the paracolpium. The medial aspect of the fourth space that extends caudally represents the paracolpium, while its lateral aspect represents the anterior mesoureter. The paracolpium, when separated from the posterior layer of Okabayashi, appears to be similar to the lateral vaginal tissue (Fig. 2.30). This procedure involves initially severing the vesicovaginal and rectovaginal ligaments and then separating the vesicovaginal and rectovaginal septa. By strongly pulling the uterus cranially, the fourth space can be extended in the direction indicated by the red arrow in panel (**a**) of Fig. 3.29. Histologically, it has been demonstrated in Fig. 4.38 that the paracolpium can be relatively easily dissected and separated from the paracystium and paraproctium in a direction along the yellow arrows.

Panel (**a**) of Fig. 4.40 depicts the paracolpium exposed after excavation and clamped with forceps. Panel (**b**) shows a schematic illustration of panel (**a**). In this case, after this photograph was taken, the superior vesical vein was excised. As anatomically demonstrated in Fig. 3.18, excavation of the fourth space can be carried out down to the pelvic floor. However, it is not required for NSRH.

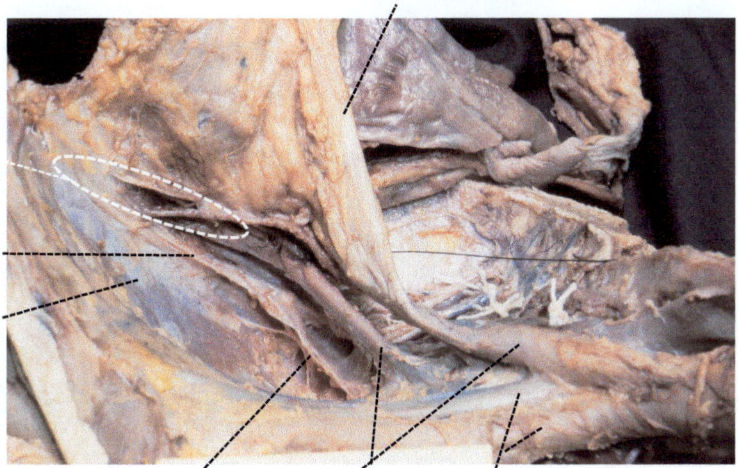

Fig. 4.37 Fixed cadaveric dissection showing the paracolpium and levator ani muscle
This photograph shows SS and pelvic floor from the perspective of the left paravesical space, corresponding to the findings shown in Fig. 4.36. Please also refer to Fig. 3.7. The anterior and posterior fasciae of the area surrounding the internal iliac vessels have been removed with the superior levator fascia excised, exposing the levator ani muscle (panel (**b**) of Fig. 2.9). The tendinous arch of the pelvic fascia extends from the pubis and attaches to the ischial spine along with the sacrospinous ligament and coccygeus muscle, the latter two forming the base of SS, or P&A's Mackenrodt ligament

As with the paravesical space, the fourth space is one that is filled with areolar connective tissue, which is conjectured to be significant for the formation of the parturient canal. The paracolpium is considered to be a pathway for vessels and nerves from the uterus, extending to the caudal end of CL of Savage/Kocks. The white dashed rectangle in panel (**a**) of Fig. 4.40 corresponds to the histological tissue specimen in panel (**c**) of Fig. 4.40. Observed here are numerous vaginal nerves with ganglia along the muscular layer and descending vascular branches.

1.20 Severance of the Vagina and Its Closure

1.20.1 Abdominal Closure

Summary and Discussion

As for the paracolpium, paracystium, and paraproctium located caudally to SS, each forms its independent longitudinal neurovascular bundle attaching parallel to the lateral aspect of its respective organ (Figs. 4.37 and 4.38). The fasciae of all three structures extend laterally, merging at the tendinous arch of the pelvic fascia, via the

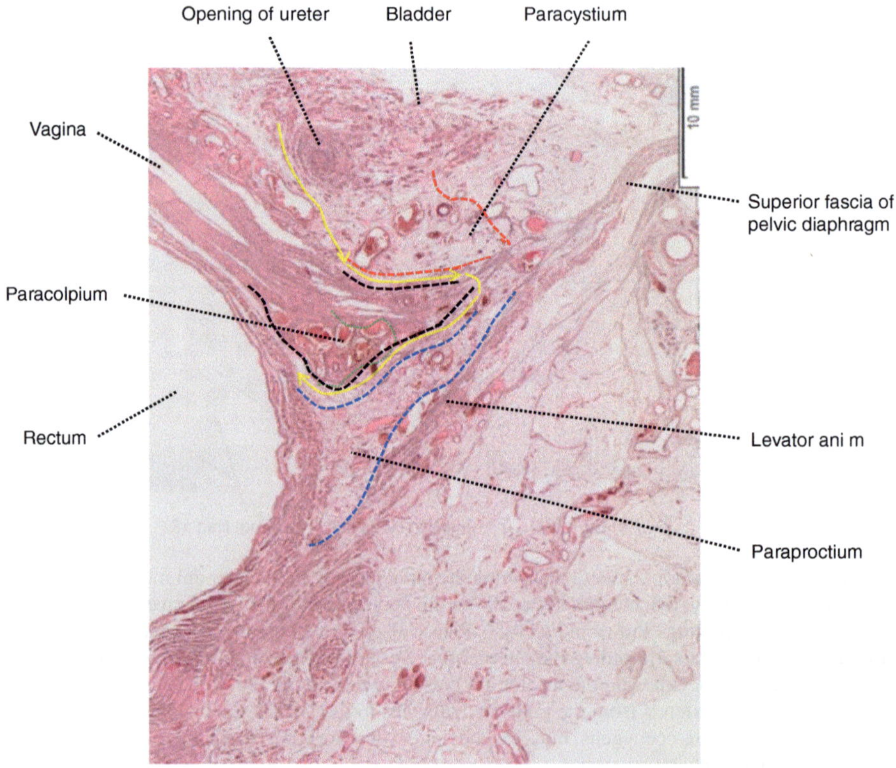

Fig. 4.38 Composition of the paravaginal tissue
This is a histological image of a frontal cross section of the uppermost part of the vagina with eosin and hematoxylin staining. The strong anterior and posterior vaginal fasciae merge at the lateral aspect of the vagina to form the paracolpium (black dashed line; see also panel (**b**) of Figs. 3.27 and 3.28). The paracolpium merges with the paracystium (red dashed line) and paraproctium (blue dashed line), all of which are similar in structure, and together, they attach to the parietal fascia, or superior levator fascia or pelvic diaphragmatic fascia, via the tendinous arch of the pelvic fascia. (Reproduced from Yabuki 2020)

Fig. 4.39 Expansion of the fourth space
Continuing from Figs. 4.25 and 4.27 on the fourth space, this surgical site in Fig. 4.39 demonstrates the fourth space expanded to the side of the vagina, extending between the paracolpium and anterior mesoureter, former of which continue from the cauterized bladder pillar. The bladder and vagina can be seen only partially excised on the right side

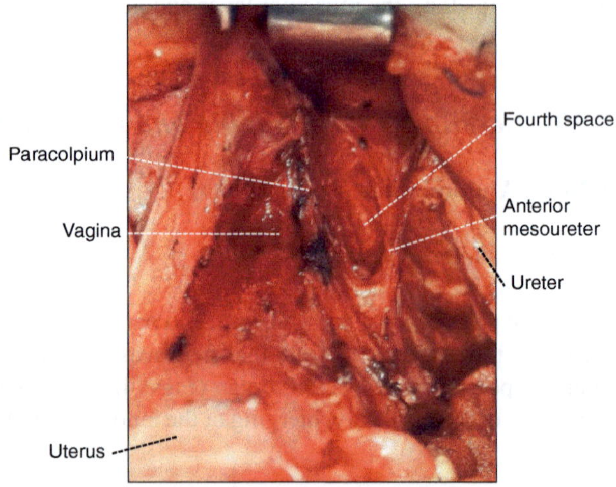

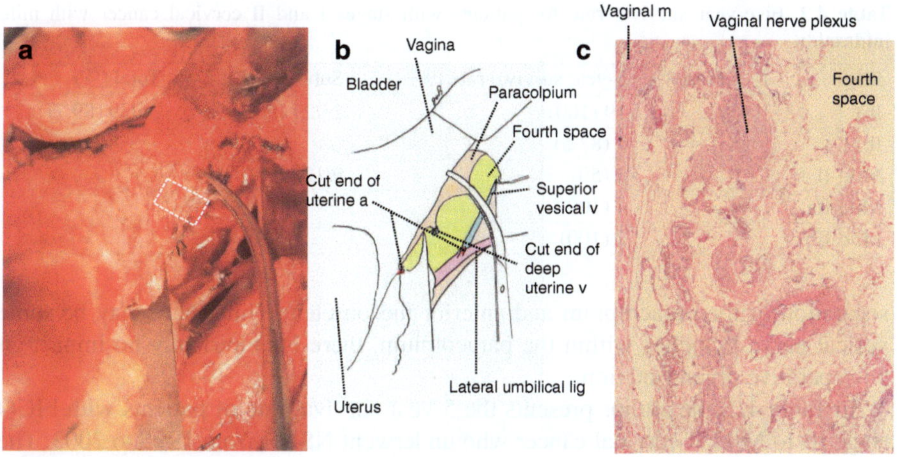

Fig. 4.40 Separation of the paracolpium with illustration and histological image
Panel (**a**) shows the paracolpium exposed by extending the fourth space and clamped with Kelly forceps. (Reproduced from Yabuki 2020)
Panel (**b**): By this manipulation, the structures can be observed from a medial aspect in the following sequence: the paracolpium, fourth space, anterior mesoureter, or superior vesical vein including vesical nerve branch, paravesical space, and lateral umbilical ligament
Panel (**c**) depicts a histological image that is stained with eosin and hematoxylin of the white rectangular area in panel (**a**). Nerves containing ganglia are observed along the muscular layer. Since the vesical nerve branches were laterally separated along with the superior vesical vein, the nerves in this specimen must be vaginal nerve branches. Please refer to Fig. 3.28. (Reproduced from Yabuki 2020)

superior fascia of the levator ani, and connecting to the tendinous arch of the levator ani (Figs. 3.27 and 4.38). In contrast, the parametrium, or *TCL*, forms a continuous transversal vascular bundle along with the vesicohypogastric fascia and lateral rectal ligament, connecting perpendicularly to the pelvic organs (Fig. 3.6). Furthermore, since the morphology and function of the uterine body, cervix, and vagina are different, it is not possible to represent each lateral ligament as having the same morphology as depicted in Fig. 2.1 by P&A and Fig. 2.3 by Yabuki. This is also schematically demonstrated in Figs. 3.30 and 3.31. Therefore, a surgical approach needed to be proposed, which would have a different anatomic perspective from that of today's for a parametrectomy and paracolpectomy. This emphasizes the necessity and importance of clinical anatomy for these procedures as well.

Creating a space between the paracolpium (dotted black line) seen in panel (**b**) of Figs. 3.27 and 4.38, paracystium (red dotted line) on its ventral aspect, and paraproctium (blue dotted line) on its dorsal aspect would result in a situation similar to that depicted from Yabuki's figure (panel (**a**) of Fig. 2.3). P&A observed this morphology in the lateral ligaments of the vagina, and the author believes that they directly applied or adapted this to the anatomy of the paracolpium.

There is a popular saying "the greater the amount of the vaginal excision, the worse the bladder paralysis." However, this issue has almost been resolved by extending the fourth space to the lateral aspect of the vagina, which allows for the

Table 4.2 Five-year survival rate for patients with stages I and II cervical cancer with mild infiltration

Stage	Cases	5-year survival rate (%)	Subtotal (%)	Total (%)
Ib1	19	19 (100)	26/27 (96.2)	35/39 (89.7)
Ib2	8	7 (87.5)		
Mild-II	6	3 (50)	9/12 (75.0)	
Mild-IIa	4	4 (100)		
Mild-IIb	2	2 (100)		

separation of the paracolpium and anterior mesoureter. While there may be some vesical nerve branches within the paracolpium, there is empirically no impact on postoperative organ function.

In Table 4.2, the author presents the 5-year survival rate of patients with FIGO stage IB to Mild II cervical cancer who underwent NSRH from 1995 to 2003. The results were obtained from a prospective study without employing an RCT. The author prefers precise surgical procedure to analytical methods when evaluating the effect of surgery.

In 2024, Plante et al. (2024) employed type II surgery in their RH, which was published in N Engl J Med titled: Simple versus radical hysterectomy in women with low-risk cervical cancer. This type II surgery, which corresponds to Class II in Piver classification and type B in Q&M classification, was adopted for classification by the European Organization for Research and Treatment of Cancer-Gynecological Cancer Group (EORTC-GCG) (Verleye et al. 2009). These surgical procedures are equivalent to the Wertheim procedure. Although the definition of RH may not be clear, a factor essential to RH, which is common practice worldwide, encompasses total excision of the lateral parametrium. This is understandable considering the historical development of RH including a dialogue between Wertheim and Mackenrodt (Mackenrodt criticizes us claiming that due to the application of these clamps, more parametrium is left on the pelvic floor. We cannot agree to this as happily, these clamps can be very closely applied on the pelvic floor.) and excision of TCL including the lateral rectal ligament by L&S (Latzko and Schiffmann 1919)/ Okabayashi (1921; Okabayashi 1952) in 1921/Meigs (1954), and NSRH by Yabuki et al. (1991, 1996, 2000; Yabuki 1997) in 1991 and 1996 as well as the latter's non-excision of the lateral rectal ligament and preservation of the vesical nerve branches. From such a perspective, it is doubtful to term the Wertheim procedure and/or modified Wertheim procedure as an RH. Moreover, the surgical procedure Ramirez et al. (2018) employed was type II or III RH according to the Piver classification, which was published in N Engl J Med in 2018. Piver class II corresponds to the Wertheim procedure, and Piver class III is clearly described as the Meigs procedure (Meigs 1954). The Meigs procedure must be the one published in his surgical manual in 1954 and corresponds to the Latzko/Okabayashi procedure with a description of the lateral rectal ligament excision, which is accompanied with an illustration (panel (**b**) of Fig. 2.8). Evaluating the outcome of the Wertheim and Meigs procedure as being comparable cannot be called evidence-based medicine even if RCT is employed for their analyses.

One of the reasons why confusion arose over these surgical procedures is possibly that, in the West, only the Meigs procedure, or Latzko/Okabayashi procedure, and Wertheim procedure or modified Wertheim procedure have existed as routinely conducted surgery for cancer of the uterine cervix. According to a report by Mangler (Mangler et al. 2013) in 2012, 71.7% of RH consisted of the Wertheim procedure and 13.7% TMMR. Trials undertaken by Ramirez, et al. began in 2008 and by Plante et al. in 2012. In these cases, it was natural to choose the Wertheim procedure, avoiding the risky Meigs procedure, when a combined treatment by chemoradiotherapy was available (Morris et al. 1999; Rose et al. 1999). An appraisal was given by Raspagliesi, et al. (Range and Woodburne 1964) in 2004 of the author's NSRH that was cited in 2005 (Sakuragi et al. 2005) and 2007 (Fujii et al. 2007). This may be the reason why, in the West, the author's surgical procedure around 2010 still existed only in the literature, not becoming well known and introduced into practice. The Wertheim or modified Wertheim procedure is undoubtedly feasible for tumors with lesions measuring no more than 2 cm. However, in invasive carcinoma with 2018 FIGO Staging for IB3, a clear distinction is required to be made for a semi-RH and RH. Currently, we cannot ignore the fact that there are many people who have no choice but to rely on surgery. Moreover, there is a promising future for expansion of RH when drugs and their method of administration are further developed for efficacious treatment in cancer of the uterine cervix, especially one that infiltrates into the lymph nodes. This is the image the author has for the future of RH.

2 Extended Radical Hysterectomy and Discussion

Since 1950, the International Federation of Gynecology and Obstetrics (FIGO) has consistently not recommended targeting stage II cervical cancer (CC) for surgery (Bhatla et al. 2019). However, challenges in the twentieth century such as intraoperative hemorrhage and postoperative bladder and rectal dysfunction are largely resolved as a result of the emergence of new surgical procedures and anatomical understanding (Yabuki et al. 1991, 1996, 2000; Yabuki 1997). Certainly, surgeries like Latzko's, Okabayashi's, and Meigs' in the twentieth century carried risks such as hemorrhage and bladder paralysis. However, speaking from the experience of having carried out the Okabayashi procedure and finally challenged it with successful results, the author (Yabuki 2007, 2016, 2019, 2020, 2023; Yabuki et al. 1996, 2000, 2005, 2011) believes that FIGO's assessment is rather negative toward the advancements in current RH. Undoubtedly, speaking from the perspective of litigation, the risks associated with surgery are high. However, when it comes to the long-term sequelae of today's successful surgery for patients with cervical cancer, aside from the psychological aspect of losing the uterus, the residual effects are relatively minor compared to those of side effects from radiation that may persist or emerge even after 20 years. It cannot be said at this time that the effectiveness of chemotherapy has reached the same level as that of surgical treatment. However, there are high expectations in the future for the use of these therapeutic drugs

(Bhatla et al. 2019; Angioli et al. 2012; Topalian et al. 2015; Schumacher and Schreiber 2015; Dunn et al. 2002; Tewari et al. 2014), which are showing remarkable progress but not without significant side effects. To reduce complications and enhance effectiveness of treatment, combinations of various treatment modalities should be considered and tried rather than relying solely on monotherapy. If surgery is restricted to stage I cervical cancer as FIGO suggests, there will be no progress in new surgical techniques. To effectively utilize anticancer agents that are to be developed in the future, combining them with surgery is one approach. When people are diagnosed with cancer, their first utmost concern is whether surgery is a possibility. Even today, it is unthinkable when a diagnosis of cancer is given to ignore surgery as a treatment option, especially when it comes to cervical cancer. Concurrent therapy involving surgery, radiation, and anticancer agents must be studied from various perspectives, especially with the emergence of new therapeutics so as to understand the full potential of these treatment modalities.

Since the 1980s, results have begun to appear on intra-arterial chemotherapy that is primarily centered around cisplatin used for bulky tumors in FIGO stage IIB, III, and IVA cervical cancer, which has resulted in commencement of concomitant neoadjuvant intra-arterial chemotherapy and radiotherapy (Key et al. 1999; Carlson et al. 1981; Scarabelli et al. 1987; Tsubamoto et al. 2013; Patton Jr et al. 1991; Morris et al. 1995; Sueyama et al. 1995; Toita et al. 1997). Furthermore, reports on clinical trials combining RH with neoadjuvant intra-arterial chemotherapy have also been conducted. However, currently, anticipated improvement in prognosis has not been observed (Angioli et al. 2012; Katsumata et al. 2013; Eddy et al. 2007) but, looking from a different perspective, there is a possibility of success.

Since 1991, the author has conducted trials on neoadjuvant intra-arterial chemotherapy for advanced cervical cancer. The objective was to evaluate the combination of effective drug delivery methods with reduction surgery for extended RH and NSRH (Fig. 4.43). Consequently, the author carried out a surgical plan focused on FIGO stage II cervical cancer with severe infiltration. Neoadjuvant chemotherapy was administered by intra-arterial infusion of cisplatin via the internal iliac artery combined with postoperative radiotherapy. Furthermore, while considering complete recovery together with QOL, an attempt was made to carry out the procedure of non-excision of the lateral rectal ligament together with partially incorporated NSRH (Fig. 4.43).

Although MRI equipment was introduced to the author's hospital in 1993, at that time, MRI findings were only used as an adjunctive diagnostic tool for staging purposes. Furthermore, if stage II was diagnosed, no plan was forwarded for detailed investigation into the relationship between tumor size and prognosis. The author's trial spanned a period of more than 10 years during which time many technological advancements were made as well as the maturation of the surgeons' skills. Data was compiled from the results of this clinical trial that explored the potential of concomitant therapy involving drugs, surgery, and radiation.

Patients with severely advanced stage II CC were divided into two types based on FIGO stages IIA2 and IIB, which was stipulated in 2008, with their prognosis being observed.

2.1 Severely Advanced Stage IIB, or α-Type, Cervical Cancer

On pelvic examination, the carcinoma is seen to extend beyond the cervix but does not reach the pelvic wall. In other words, there is a free space between the tumor and pelvic wall. The surgical procedure for this stage is called lateral extended RH (LERH) and was combined with neoadjuvant intra-arterial chemotherapy.

2.2 Severely Advanced Stage IIA, or β-Type, Cervical Cancer

In this case, the carcinoma did not infiltrate to the lower third of the vagina. However, it infiltrated into one or more of the following nearby tissues: parametrium, paracolpium, adventitia of the bladder, rectal adventitia, vesicouterine ligament, and sacro-/rectouterine ligaments. However, the diagnosis showed that there was no infiltration into the muscular layer, and infiltration to TCL did not exceed half. The surgical procedure carried out in this case is called central extended RH (CERH) and was combined with neoadjuvant intra-arterial chemotherapy.

2.3 Methods and Results

Using Seldinger's technique for both of these surgical procedures, a catheter was inserted into the uterine artery, if possible, at its origin, administrating cisplatin or carboplatin and peplomycin sulfate, or *PEP*, each in 100 ml of saline solution (Fig. 3.25) The drugs are administered as a single-shot infusion over a period of at least 10 min, and the treatment is carried out either once or, if twice, with a 4-week interval in-between administration (Table 4.3).

The clinical response to chemotherapy was primarily assessed through internal examination and visual inspection, together with contrast-enhanced CT or MRI used as a reference. Patients with a partial response or more positive response to chemotherapy underwent surgery. In addition, external irradiation was carried out postoperatively. The irradiation dose was up to 50 Gy for a whole pelvic field without a center shield.

Table 4.3 Treatment regimen of chemotherapy and radiotherapy for patients who had undergone lateral extended RH or central extended RH

	Cisplatin (CDDP) 50 ~ 100 mg, or carboplatin (CBDCA) 300 mg,
	Peplomycin sulfate (PEP) 10 mg
	Intra-arterial single-shot infusion 1 ~ 2 times with 4-week interval
Operation method	Lateral extended radical hysterectomy
	Central extended radical hysterectomy
Postoperative irradiation	50 Gy, no central shield

Table 4.4 Supplementary surgery to lateral or central extended RH

	α-type CC	β-type CC
	Lateral extended RH	Central extended RH
Retroperitoneoscopic Para-aortic lymph node dissection (Fig. 4.41)	7	2
Removal of lateral umbilical ligament	11	7
Removal of internal iliac artery	2	0
Removal of internal iliac artery and vein (Fig. 4.42)	1	0
Total cystectomy	2	2
Ureterostomy	2	2
Partial cystectomy	0	3
Ureteroneocystostomy	0	3
Rectectomy (Figs. 4.43 and 4.44)	0	2
Total colpectomy	0	1

Additional surgeries carried out in conjunction with RH are presented in Table 4.4.

Endoscopic surgery, or left extraperitoneal approach, for paracaval and para-aortic lymph node dissection (Ando and Kanno 2023; Trimble et al. 2015) was introduced in the year 2000 (Fig. 4.41). Before the year 2000, only lymph node sampling was carried out, so those cases were excluded from the statistics.

Figure 4.42 shows removal of the internal iliac artery and vein.

Also, partial preservation of the inferior hypogastric plexus was conducted. A rectectomy with lateral dissection is shown in Fig. 4.43 with the method of its preservation illustrated in Fig. 4.44.

The assessment of these outcomes was compared to those of patients who had undergone radiotherapy, but no RCT was carried out. Perioperative information on these patients is presented in Table 4.5. By the use of pTNM classification, the difficulty of accurately determining a diagnosis for preoperative staging is demonstrated.

The 5-year overall survival rate is presented in Table 4.6 and Fig. 4.45.

The clear difference between the 21.4% survival rate for α-type cervical cancer and 66.7% for β-type cervical cancer was astounding, in which FIGO staging of the year 2009 classification was applied, but to some degree, this result was understandable, for 85.7% of α-type cervical cancer represented stage IIIC when FIGO staging in the year 2018 classification was applied. Nevertheless, the effectiveness of β-type cervical cancer treatment was believed to be due to low lymph node metastasis and direct high concentration of drugs through intra-arterial administration. This fact suggests that further examination of the relationship with the lymph flow of the vagina is required, and also the reason why there is low infiltration and/or metastasis to the vesicouterine ligament (Kraima et al. 2014).

The author is empirically convinced that, if drugs and administration methods with high therapeutic efficacy against pelvic lymph node metastases are developed, the opportunities for surgical therapy will increase. According to Plante et al.'s

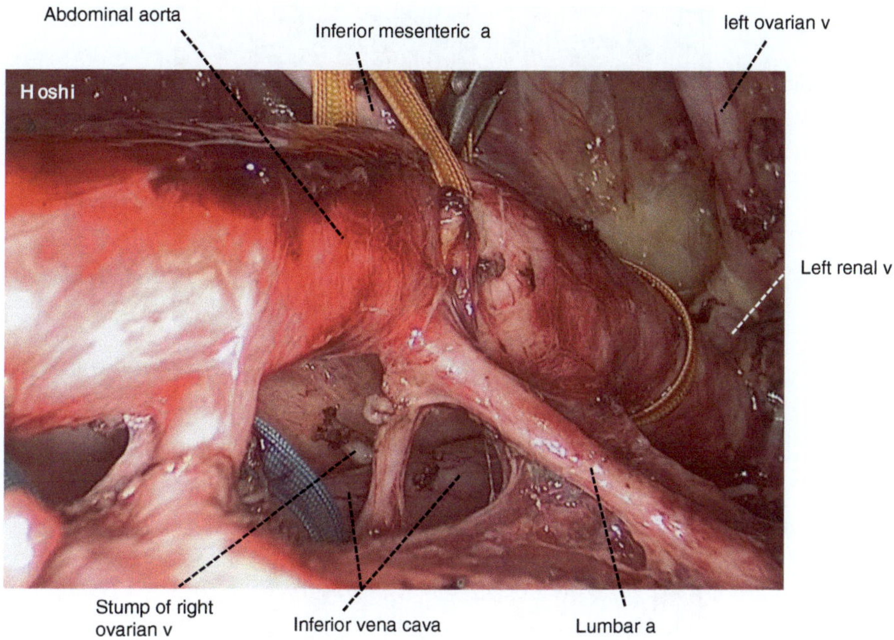

Fig. 4.41 Suspension of the abdominal aorta
The abdominal aorta is seen suspended by yellow vascular tape, and the inferior mesenteric artery is isolated from the mid-superior aspect. The inferior vena cava can be seen passing under the blue vascular tape, and, on its right, the stump of the right ovarian vein. Further, the left ovarian vein joining the left renal vein is indicated in the right upper corner. This procedure completes the dissection of the interaortocaval region. (By courtesy of Tsutomu Hoshiba, MD, PhD., my most capable and trustworthy colleague)

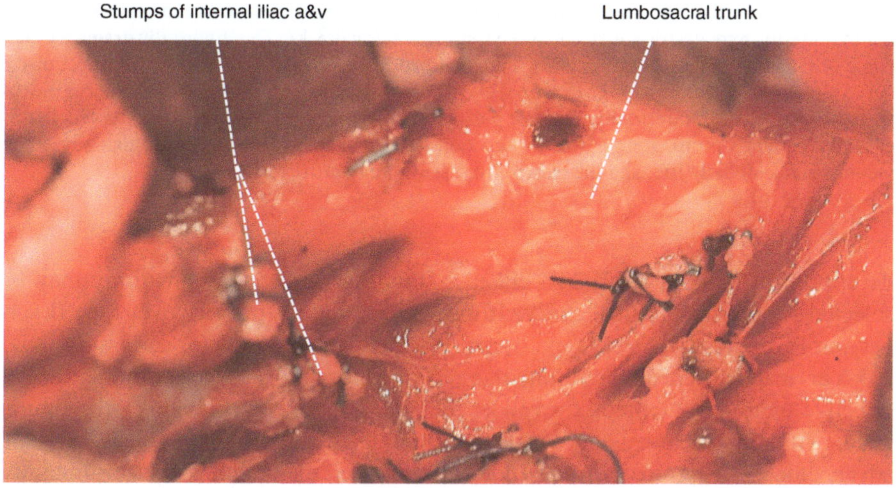

Fig. 4.42 Excision of the anterior trunks of the internal iliac vessels
The anterior trunks of the internal iliac artery/vein were excised where the inferior vesical artery/vein branches off, exposing the lumbosacral nerve trunk leaving a pocket-like excision scar. This case involved the excision of the deep external iliac lymph nodes

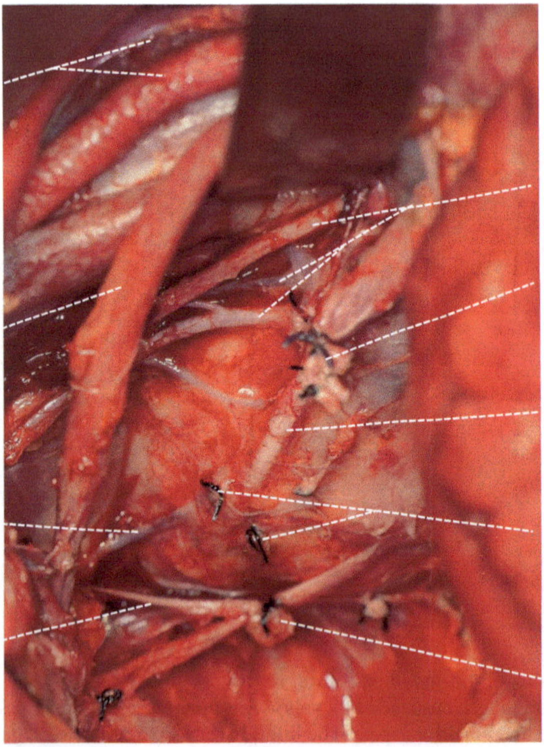

Fig. 4.43 Nerve-sparing radical hysterectomy and rectectomy (NSRH)
This shows a total mesorectal excision carried out with lateral dissection together with an RH on a patient where the cancerous tumor had invaded the rectal adventitia. The photograph also shows the right parietal stump of SS. In Fig. 4.44, the lateral rectal ligament is divided into medial and lateral portions by the inferior hypogastric plexus. The middle rectal vessels can be seen penetrating the inferior hypogastric plexus also seen in Figs. 3.7 and 3.17. This figure illustrates the outcome of excision of the lateral rectal ligament and an RH carried out on the lateral aspect of the nerve plexus. A rectectomy by TME was also carried out on the medial aspect of the nerve plexus with the rectal nerves, inferior hypogastric plexus, and its vesical branches being preserved. In this case, the patient's postoperative bladder function was maintained within a range that caused no inconvenience to daily life, and the patient lived for more than 10 years

description (Plante et al. 2024), either a simple or radical hysterectomy may be selected for uterine cervical cancer if the former is given priority over type II surgery, or Piver class II, Q&M type B, and Wertheim procedures, for early-stage low-risk cervical cancer. In addition, there is the possibility of developing further effective treatment methods for cancer that can be utilized now and in the future. Also, with improvements in surgical technique, including robotic surgery, and advancements in cytotoxic drugs, molecular targeted therapeutics, cancer immunotherapy drugs, and other new therapeutic agents, further advanced combination treatments will be developed.

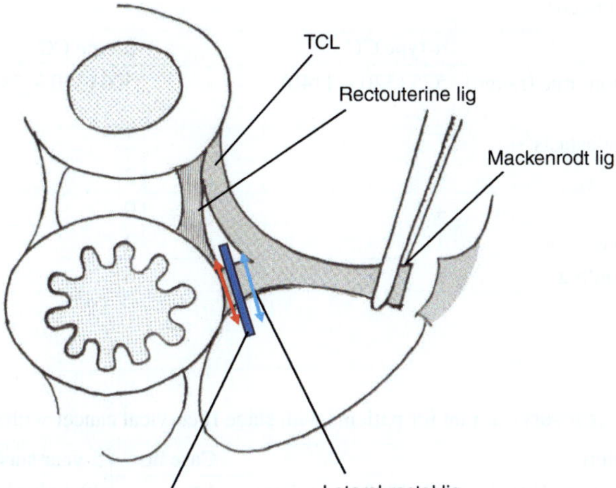

Fig. 4.44 Schematic illustration showing excision of the lateral rectal ligament in nerve-sparing surgery
Seen in this figure, TME is carried out on the medial aspect of the red double-headed arrow, while lateral dissection of the lateral rectal ligament is carried out on the lateral aspect of the blue double-headed arrow

Table 4.5 Perioperative data on patients who had undergone lateral or central extended RH

	α-type CC	β-type CC
Number of patients	14	9
Trial period	1993 ~ 2002	1990 ~ 2002
Median age of patients (range)	53 (32 ~ 74)	60 (31 ~ 70)
Histologic type		
Squamous cell carcinoma	10	8
Adenocarcinoma	2	1
Adenosquamous carcinoma	2	0
Response to chemotherapy		
Complete response	2	2
Partial response	12	6
No change	1	1
Progressive disease	0	0
pTNM classification		
pT2	8	5
pT3	4	2
pT4	2	2
Median intraoperative blood loss (range) (ml)	1120 (3960 ~ 615)	1850 (770 ~ 2440)

Table 4.5 (continued)

	α-type CC	β-type CC
Median operation time (range) (min)	525 (320 ~ 1140)	500 (340 ~ 784)
Lymph node metastasis		
N1	8	2
M1	4	0
Local recurrence	11	2
Spontaneous voiding	8	6

Table 4.6 Five-year survival rate for patients with stage II cervical cancer with severe infiltration

Surgical procedure		Case no	5-year survival rate (%)	
Extended RH with ia-NACT (1990–2002)	LERH	14	39.1 (9/23)	21.4 (3/14)
	CERH	9		66.7 (6/9)

ia-NACT intra-arterial neoadjuvant chemotherapy, *LERH* lateral extended RH, *CERH* central extended RH

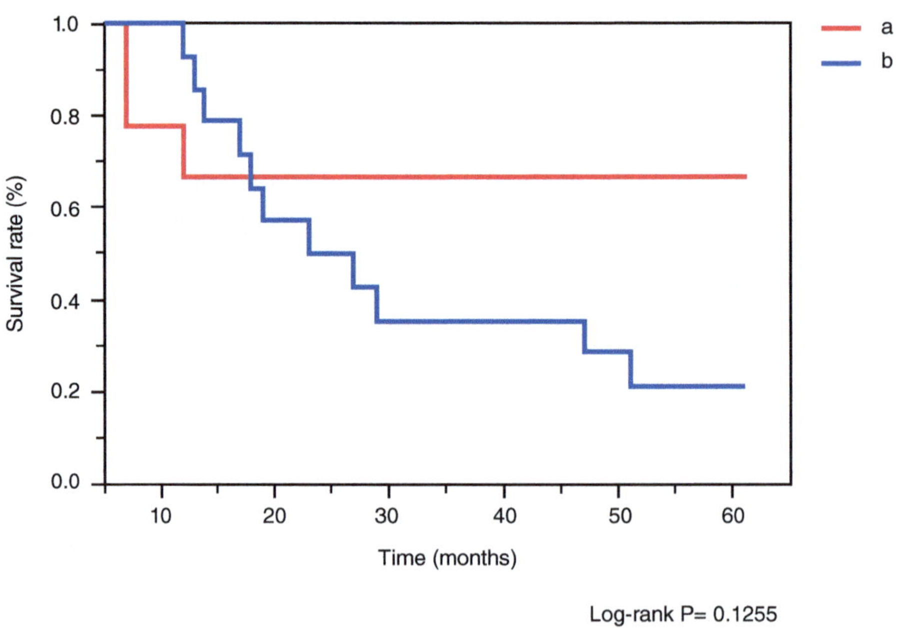

Fig. 4.45 The Kaplan-Meier survival curve showing overall survival rates following super-radical hysterectomy. (**a**) Central extended super-RH, (**b**) Lateral extended super-RH

References

Ando M, Kanno K (2023) Gynecological endoscopic surgery: Kurashiki method. Chūgai-Igakusha, Tokyo. (in Japanese)

Angioli R, Plotti F, Montera R et al (2012) Neoadjuvant chemotherapy plus radical surgery followed by chemotherapy in locally advanced cervical cancer. Gynecol Oncol. https://doi.org/10.1016/j.ygyno.2012.07.104. PMID: 22819938. Clinical Trial

Averette HE, Nguyen HN, Donato DM et al (1993) Radical hysterectomy for invasive cervical cancer: a 25-year prospective experience with the Miami technique. Cancer Suppl 71:1422–1437. PMID: 8431876. https://doi.org/10.1002/cncr.2820710407

Bhatla N, Berk JS, Cuello FM et al (2019) Revised FIGO staging for carcinoma of the cervix uteri. Int J Gynaecol Obstet 145:129–135

Campbell RM (1950) Anatomy and histology of the sacrouterine ligament. Am J Obstet Gynecol 59:1–12. PMID: 15399622. https://doi.org/10.1016/0002-9378(50)90334-6

Carlson JA, Freedman RS, Wallace S et al (1981) Intraarterial cis-platinum in the management of squamous cell carcinoma of the uterine cervix. Gynecol Oncol 12:92–98. PMID: 6168518. https://doi.org/10.1016/0090-8258(81)90100-1

Drake RL, Vogl W, Mitchell AWM (eds) (2005) Gray's Anatomy for Students. Elsevier, Philadelphia

Dunn GP, Bruce AT, Ikeda H et al (2002) Cancer immunoediting: from immunosurveillance to tumor escape. Nat Immunol 3:991–998. PMID: 12407406. https://doi.org/10.1038/ni1102-991

Eddy GL, Bundy BN, Creasman WT et al (2007) Treatment of ("bulky") stage IB cervical cancer with or without neoadjuvant vincristine and cisplatin prior to radical hysterectomy and pelvic/para-aortic lymphadenectomy: a phase III trial of the gynecologic oncology group. Gynecol Oncol 106:362–369. PMID: 17493669. https://doi.org/10.1016/j.ygyno.2007.04.007

Fujii S, Takakura K, Matsumura N et al (2007) Anatomic identification and functional outcomes of the nerve sparing Okabayashi radical hysterectomy. Gynecol Oncol 107(1):4–13. PMID: 17905140. https://doi.org/10.1016/j.ygyno.2007.08.076

Höckel M, Horn LC, Fritsch H (2005) Association between the mesenchymal compartment of uterovaginal organogenesis and local tumor spread in stage IB-IIB cervical carcinoma: a prospective study. Lancet Oncol 6:751–756. PMID: 16198980. https://doi.org/10.1016/S1470-2045(05)70324-7

Katsumata N, Yoshikawa H, Kobayashi H et al (2013) Phase III randomised controlled trial of neoadjuvant chemotherapy plus radical surgery vs radical surgery alone for stages IB2, IIA2, and IIB cervical cancer: a Japan Clinical Oncology Group trial (JCOG 0102). Br J Cancer 108(10):1957–1963. PMID: 23640393 PMCID: PMC3671094. https://doi.org/10.1038/bjc.2013.179

Key HM, Bundy BN, Stehman FB et al (1999) Cisplatin, radiation, and adjuvant hysterectomy compared with radiation and adjuvant hysterectomy for bulky stage IB cervical carcinoma. N Engl J Med 340:1154–1161. PMID: 10202166. https://doi.org/10.1056/NEJM199904153401503

Kraima AC, Derks M, Smit NN et al (2014) Lymphatic drainage pathways from the cervix uteri: implications for radical hysterectomy? Gynecol Oncol 132(1):107–113. PMID: 24201016. https://doi.org/10.1016/j.ygyno.2013.10.030

Latzko W, Schiffmann J (1919) Zur Radikaloperation des Gebarmutterkrebses. 361 Diskussinsbemerkungen. Zbl Gynäk 43:689–698

Mangler M, Zech N, Schneider A et al (2013) Aspects of therapy for cervical cancer in Germany 2012: results from a survey of German gynaecological hospitals. Geburtshilfe Frauenheilkd 73(3):227–238. PMID: 24771915, PMCID: PMC3964377. https://doi.org/10.1055/s-0032-1328302

Meigs JV (1954) Radical hysterectomy with bilateral dissection of the pelvic lymph nodes. In: Meigs JV (ed) Surgical treatment of cancer of the cervix. Grune Stratton, New York, pp 149–216

Morris M, Eifel PJ, Burke TW et al (1995) Treatment of locally advanced cervical cancer with concurrent radiation and intra-arterial chemotherapy. Gynecol Oncol 57:72–78. PMID: 7705704. https://doi.org/10.1006/gyno.1995.1101

Morris M, Eifel PJ, Lu J et al (1999) Pelvic radiation with concurrent chemotherapy compared with pelvic and para-aortic radiation for high-risk cervical cancer. N Engl J Med 340:1137–1143. https://doi.org/10.1056/NEJM199904153401501. PMID: 10202164

Okabayashi H (1921) Radical abdominal hysterectomy for cancer of cervix uteri. Surg Gynecol Obstet 33:335–341

Okabayashi H (1952) Systematic abdominal radical hysterectomy for cancer of cervix uteri. Kanehara, Tokyo. (in Japanese)

Patton TJ Jr, Kavanagh JJ, Delclos L et al (1991) Five-year survival in patients given intra-arterial chemotherapy prior to radiotherapy for advanced squamous carcinoma of the cervix and vagina. Gynecol Oncol 42:54–59. PMID: 1916511. https://doi.org/10.1016/0090-8258(91)90230-3

Peham HV, Amreich J (1930) Gynäkologische Operationslehre. VERLAG VON S. KARGER, BASEL

Plante M, Kwon JS, Ferguson S, Samouëlian V, Ferron G et al (2024) Simple versus radical hysterectomy in women with low-risk cervical cancer. N Engl J Med 390:819–829. https://doi.org/10.1056/NEJMoa2308900

Ramirez PT, Frumovitz M, Pareja R et al (2018) Minimally invasive versus abdominal radical hysterectomy for cervical cancer. N Engl J Med 379:1895–1904. PMID: 30380365. https://doi.org/10.1056/NEJMoa1806395

Range RL, Woodburne RT (1964) The gross and microscopic anatomy of the transverse cervical ligament. Am J Obstet Gynecol 90:460–467. PMID: 14217646. https://doi.org/10.1016/0002-9378(64)90802-6

Reiffenstuhl G (1964) The lymphatics of the female organs. JB Lippincott, Philadelphia

Rose PG, Bundy BN, Watkins EB et al (1999) Concurrent cisplatin-based radiotherapy and chemotherapy for locally advanced cervical cancer. N Engl J Med 340:1144–1153. PMID: 10202165. https://doi.org/10.1056/NEJM199904153401502

Sakuragi N, Todo Y, Kudo M et al (2005) A systematic nerve-sparing radical hysterectomy technique in invasive cervical cancer for preserving postsurgical bladder function. Int J Gynecol Cancer 15(2):389–397. PMID: 15823132. https://doi.org/10.1111/j.1525-1438.2005.15236.x

Scarabelli C, Tumolo S, De Paoli A et al (1987) Intermittent pelvic arterial infusion with peptichemio, doxorubicin, and cisplatin for locally advanced and recurrent carcinoma of the uterine cervix. Cancer 60:25–30. PMID: 3581031. https://doi.org/10.1002/1097-0142(19870701)60:1<25:aid-cncr2820600106>3.0.co;2-5

Schumacher TN, Schreiber RD (2015) Neoantigens in cancer immunotherapy. Science 348(6230):69–74. PMID: 25838375. https://doi.org/10.1126/science.aaa4971

Sueyama H, Nakano M, Sakumoto K et al (1995) Intra-arterial chemotherapy with cisplatin followed by radical radiotherapy for locally advanced cervical cancer. Gynecol Oncol 59(3):327–332. https://doi.org/10.1006/gyno.1995.9968

Tewari KS, Sill MW, Long H 3rd et al (2014) Improved survival with bevacizumab in advanced cervical cancer. N Engl J Med 370:734–743. PMID: 24552320, PMCID: PMC4010094. https://doi.org/10.1056/NEJMoa1309748

Toita T, Sakumoto K, Higashi M et al (1997) Therapeutic value of neoadjuvant intra-arterial chemotherapy (cisplatin) and irradiation for locally advanced uterine cervical cancer. Gynecol Oncol 65:421–424. PMID: 9190968. https://doi.org/10.1006/gyno.1997.4702

Topalian SL, Drake CG, Pardoll DM (2015) Immune checkpoint blockade: a common denominator approach to cancer therapy. Cancer Cell 27:450–461. PMID: 25858804, PMCID: PMC4400238. https://doi.org/10.1016/j.ccell.2015.03.001

Trimble CL, Morrow MP, Kraynyak KA et al (2015) Safety, efficacy, and immunogenicity of VGX-3100, a therapeutic synthetic DNA vaccine targeting human papillomavirus 16 and 18 E6 and E7 proteins for cervical intraepithelial neoplasia 2/3: a randomised, double-blind, placebo-controlled phase 2b trial. Lancet 386(10008):2078–2088. https://doi.org/10.1016/S0140-6736(15)00239-1. PMID: 26386540, PMC4888059

Tsubamoto H, Maeda H, Kanazawa R et al (2013) Phase II trial on neoadjuvant intravenous and trans-uterine arterial chemotherapy for locally advanced bulky cervical adenocarcinoma. Gynecol Oncol 129:129–134. PMID: 23333929. https://doi.org/10.1016/j.ygyno.2013.01.007

Verleye I, Vergot I, Reed N et al (2009) Quality assurance for radical hysterectomy for cervical cancer: the view of the European Organization for Research and Treatment of Cancer-Gynecological Cancer Group (EORTC-GCG). Ann Oncol 20:1631–1638

Yabuki Y (1997) Cardinal ligament dissection based on a new theory. CEM J Gynecol Oncol 2:278–287. [Google Scholar]

Yabuki Y (2007) Anatomy of the pelvis for radical hysterectomy: does extensive resection of the vagina result in severer bladder dysfunction? The 16th Annual Review Course on Gynecologic Oncology and Pathology. Kyoto, Japan

Yabuki Y (2016) Clinical anatomy of the subserous layer: an amalgamation of gross and clinical anatomy. Clin Anat 29:508–515

Yabuki Y (2019) New radical hysterectomy for uterine cancer. In: Theory and technique for nerve-sparing operation, 3rd edn. Medical View, Tokyo. (in Japanese with figure legend in English)

Yabuki Y (2020) Twenty-first century radical hysterectomy: journey from descriptive to practical anatomy. Gynecol Oncol Rep 34:100623. https://doi.org/10.1016/j.gore.2020.100623. PMID: 32984492, PMCID: PMC7498749

Yabuki Y (2023) Two lateral parametria in radical hysterectomy: history and outcome. J Obstet Gynecol Res 43:1069–1078. https://doi.org/10.1111/jog.15559

Yabuki Y, Asamoto A, Hoshiba T et al (1991) Dissection of the cardinal ligament in radical hysterectomy for cervical cancer with emphasis on the lateral ligament. Am J Obstet Gynecol 164:7–14. PMID: 1986630. https://doi.org/10.1016/0002-9378(91)90614-w

Yabuki Y, Asamoto A, Hoshiba T et al (1996) A new proposal for radical hysterectomy. Gynecol Oncol 62:370–378. PMID: 8812535. [PubMed]. https://doi.org/10.1006/gyno.1996.0251

Yabuki Y, Asamoto A, Hoshiba T et al (2000) Radical hysterectomy: an anatomic evaluation of parametrial dissection. Gynecol Oncol 77:155–163. https://doi.org/10.1006/gyno.1999. PMID: 10739705

Yabuki Y et al (2005) Discrepancies between classic anatomy and modern gynecologic surgery on pelvic connective tissue structure: harmonization of those concepts by collaborative cadaver dissection. Am J Obstet Gynecol 193:7–15

Yabuki Y, Murakami G, Hoshiba T et al (2011) Redefinition of the pelvic connective tissue: in-situ histologic examination. Female Pelvic Med Reconstr Surg 17:60–66

Correction to: Nerve-Sparing Radical Hysterectomy

Correction to:
Chapters 2 and 4 in: Y. Yabuki, *Nerve-Sparing Radical Hysterectomy*, https://doi.org/10.1007/978-981-96-7194-6

This book was recently published. The attached corrections are to be updated in the below listed chapters as mentioned below:

1. Chapter 2- Figure 2.30 in Page 47, to the position of the blue circle (please refer to the PPT).
2. Chapter 4- The abbreviation of Vesicouterine Ligament in Page 111, should be updated to VUL.

Current output:

1. Figure 2.30 in Chapter 2, Page 47
2. Excision of the Vesicouterine Ligament (**TCL**) (Chapter 4, Page 111)

Required Output:

1. Figure 2.30 in Chapter 2, Page 47

The updated version of these chapters can be found at
https://doi.org/10.1007/978-981-96-7194-6_2
https://doi.org/10.1007/978-981-96-7194-6_4

Y. Yabuki, *Nerve-Sparing Radical Hysterectomy*,
https://doi.org/10.1007/978-981-96-7194-6_5

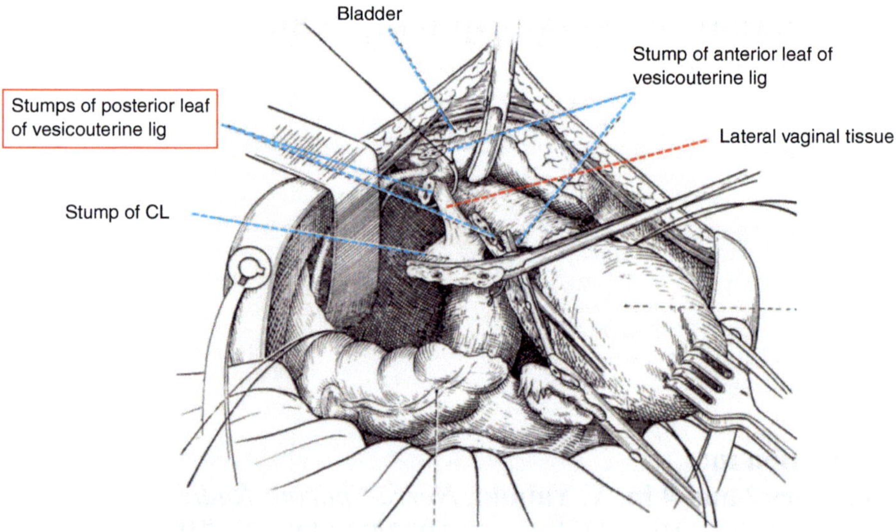

2. Excision of the Vesicouterine Ligament **(VUL)** (Chapter 4, Page 111)

Postscript

The author embarked upon writing this book on surgery by combining the content of his nine English-written articles published between 1980 and 2023 together with his photographic images taken during surgery and cadaveric dissections. The author takes pride in having taken part in the reshaping of the 100-year-old history of surgery for cervical cancer inherited from L&S since 1919 into a present-day QOL-oriented surgery focused on anatomy, surgical techniques, and functional preservation. Specifically, he is confident and proud in his newly established theories and surgical techniques and new definitions given in 1991 for TCL and the vesicouterine ligament, together with discovery of nerve-sparing surgery in 1996, and its application to laparoscopic surgery in 2000. Moreover, the warm clarity and three-dimensional color of his photographic images captured with a Nikon lens (Medical-Nikkor 120 mm) are unmatched by current digital images with the author's intention to also preserve these images for future generations.

Y. Yabuki, *Nerve-Sparing Radical Hysterectomy*,
https://doi.org/10.1007/978-981-96-7194-6

MIX
Papier aus verantwortungsvollen Quellen
Paper from responsible sources
FSC® C105338

If you have any concerns about our products,
you can contact us on
ProductSafety@springernature.com

In case Publisher is established outside the EU,
the EU authorized representative is:
Springer Nature Customer Service Center GmbH
Europaplatz 3, 69115 Heidelberg, Germany

Printed by Libri Plureos GmbH
in Hamburg, Germany